BIRTH CONTROL MASTERY: A COMPREHENSIVE PRACTICAL GUIDE TO UNDERSTANDING BIRTH CONTROL METHODS AND SIDE EFFECTS ON THE BRAIN AND BODY

The Science Behind a Women's Body, Hormone Balancing, Fertility Signs, Natural and Medical Ways of Birth Prevention

GABRIELLE TOWNSEND

Silk Publishing

Contents

Introduction

Contraceptives save the lives of mothers and newborns. Contraceptives also reduce abortion. As a result of contraceptive use, there were 26 million fewer unsafe abortions in the world's poorest countries in just one year, according to the most recent data.

Melinda Gates

The need for birth control is often common among those who wish to prevent pregnancy for one reason or another. Thanks to civilization and science that have made it possible to have it easy when it comes to methods of birth control. Gone are the days when preventing pregnancy simply meant one thing: celibacy. You can now prevent conception with pills, devices, surgical procedures, and even natural means.

It is crucial to realize that there is no such thing as a "best" birth control method. The advantages and disadvantages of each strategy are clear. Whether or not one becomes a parent is a choice that can be made by both partners. Birth control, or contraception, isn't a simple decision to make. There is a lot to consider. In order to get started, this book will inform you and your spouse about various methods of birth control. Inquire with your doctor as well.

Your general health, your desire to start a family in the future, the effectiveness of each birth control technique, probable adverse effects, and your degree of comfort with using it are all factors to consider when choosing a method of birth control.

It's important to remember that even the most successful methods of birth control can go wrong. Your chances of getting pregnant decrease if you don't employ the procedure appropriately. Different methods of birth control are discussed in this book, as well as important considerations to keep in mind when determining whether or not to go on birth control.

There are a plethora of options for preventing pregnancy. It's best to go with the one that best suits your needs. Condoms should always be used for intercourse because most methods do not protect against STIs. While contemplating your options for contraception, ask yourself: Where can I obtain this method? How easy is the method to implement? How much does this method cost? Well, I will say you don't have to overthink any of these questions. Why? Because this book covers everything you need to prevent conception.

In this book, you are going to learn the hidden secrets about birth control, various birth control methods, the science of women's body and how to properly read your menstrual cycle to have a better understanding of your hormones and how your body works. Let's get started!

1

Understanding Birth Control

Birth control is exactly what it sounds like: a method of preventing pregnancies. Unless a woman and her partner decide to stop having children, this does not indicate that births will be stopped. Every health worker should be able to administer birth control (contraceptives) to their patients if they need it. Women die if they don't use birth control. Too many pregnancies in a short period of time weaken them, resulting in their death during childbirth. Infants die because they can't get enough breast milk.

All contemporary contraceptive methods carry some risk. Birth control and sterilization deaths are only a small proportion of the deaths caused by childbirth and illegal abortion. Nutrition, living standards, access to health-care services, and in particular parental care, as well as the availability of both voluntary sterilization and legally permissible abortion, are all important contributors to maternal mortality.

BENEFITS OF BIRTH CONTROL PILLS

There are many other benefits to using a birth control pill in addition to helping you avoid pregnancy, such as making your period less painful and more regular, improving your skin, and reducing your chance of some cancers.

A whopping 14 percent of those who use the pill do so solely for reasons other than birth control. Over half of pill users use it for non-pregnancy-related reasons, as well. Beyond avoiding conception, there are other advantages to using birth control pills.

Regular Periods

Birth control tablets might help you know exactly when your period will arrive. The estrogen and progestin hormones used in traditional birth control pills are very similar to those produced by your ovaries. "Active" tablets are taken for three weeks; then inactive pills are taken for one week. During the week you take the inactive pills, you will get your menstruation.

The use of the pills can be tailored to suit your individual needs and lifestyle, thanks to newer possibilities. A shorter monthly cycle is now possible with new products that contain 24 active pills and 4 inactive ones. Taking active pills for a longer period of time is possible with these extended-cycle versions. Before taking a break, you can try taking active tablets for three months. To put it another way: Your menstrual cycle will occur just four times every year. Avoid your period during hectic periods like final exams and sports or social events if you want. After a year of taking active pills every day for a year, you can completely stop your menstruation. Your menstruation can be reduced or eliminated with the use of another variety known as a "minipill." Every day, for a total of 28 days, you are supposed to take this pill.

2

Help With Cramps, PMS, and Anemia

By blocking ovulation and thinning the uterine lining, birth control tablets may reduce your chance of heavy monthly bleeding. Iron-deficiency anemia, which is caused by severe bleeding, can be reduced by having a lighter period. Because the pill stops ovulation and reduces the length of your menstrual cycle, it can help alleviate unpleasant cramps.

Menstrual cramps, mood swings, breast pain, weight gain, bloating, and acne can all be alleviated by birth control tablets if you suffer from PMS or PMDD (premenstrual dysphoric disorder). Menstrual migraines may be reduced or eliminated if you take the pill to regulate your hormone levels.

Relieve Endometriosis Symptoms and Prevent Ovarian Cysts

When the lining of the uterus grows outside of it, it is known as endometriosis. Menstrual cramps and severe pain are possible side effects. By eliminating your periods, birth control medications may help alleviate some of the symptoms of endometriosis. Ovarian cysts may be prevented in the future by taking the medications.

Clear Up Skin and Prevent Unwanted Hair Growth

Birth control tablets can reduce the levels of male hormones produced by your ovaries, so lowering acne and hair development in the midline of your body. Some people may have hair growth on the upper lip, chin, between the breasts, belly button and pubic bone, or down the inner thighs if their levels of these hormones are higher than normal or if they are susceptible to them. Within six months, you should notice a decrease in the amount of unwanted hair.

Help With Polycystic Ovarian Syndrome (PCOS)

Women with the polycystic ovarian syndrome (PCOS) have an imbalance of hormones in which the ovaries produce excess testosterone. Some of the side effects include acne, abnormal menstrual cycles, and hair growth. An increase in estrogen and decreased testosterone levels, as well as regular menstrual cycles, are all benefits of taking birth control pills.

Reduce Your Cancer Risk

Some malignancies are more likely to be acquired if you use birth control tablets, while others are less likely. If a woman has ever taken the pill, she has a lower risk of developing ovarian cancer by 30% to 50%. Taking it for a longer period of time reduces your risk of developing this particular form of cancer. After you stop taking the pill, the lower risk persists for up to 30 years.

Endometrial cancer is less common in women who have used birth control tablets. At the very least, it reduces your chances of developing this type of cancer by 30 percent. The lower your risk is, the longer you take the medication. After you stop taking the pill, this benefit continues to last for many years. Colorectal cancer may also be lowered while taking the tablet, according to new research findings.

It gives you the freedom to bleed on your own terms

Bleeding is an unavoidable part of being a woman during menstruation for the majority of women. There is, however, an alternative. Most birth control kits include a week's supply of hormone-free placebo tablets. There is nothing wrong with taking a tablet every day. While taking these placebo pills, you're more likely to receive your period.

Skip the placebo pills if you're planning a vacation or other event during that week. Instead, create a brand new pack from scratch. Taking monophasic birth control pills, which have the same hormone dose in each pill, is ideal for this strategy. You can skip the last week of birth control tablets in a pack. To avoid your period, you might use other techniques like IUDs and patches.

REMEMBER: Not everyone can benefit from hormonal birth control. High blood pressure and blood clots are more likely in people over 35 who smoke. Even if you're not a smoker, hormonal birth control, such as combination pills and patches, can raise your risk of blood clots and high blood pressure.

A wide range of physical and emotional side effects, ranging from joint pain to insanity, can be associated with hormonal birth control. Make sure to notify your doctor about any previous birth control adverse effects you've had.

Hormonal birth control methods do not protect against sexually transmitted illnesses. Use a condom or other kind of protection during sex unless you and your long-term partner have both been tested.

Your doctor can help you analyze the advantages and disadvantages of each treatment option to help you decide which one is best for your situation. An online tool provided by Bedsider, an organization dedicated to the prevention of unintended pregnancies, helps you to locate local providers of free or low-cost birth control.

SIDE EFFECTS OF BIRTH CONTROL PILLS

Hormone levels are altered by the use of birth control tablets, which can result in a variety of undesirable side effects. Within two to three months, these effects are normally gone. However, they can continue for longer. Oral contraceptive tablets are used by around 12.6% of American women ages 15 to 49. Most females can safely utilize them.

Changing brands or methods of birth control may be necessary if the negative effects continue for a lengthy period of time or are extremely unpleasant. Oral contraceptive adverse effects are discussed in detail in the following sections.

Spotting between periods

When vaginal bleeding occurs in between menstrual cycles, it is referred to as breakthrough bleeding or spotting. It can appear as a brown discharge or as minor bleeding. The most common adverse effect of birth control tablets is spotting or irregular periods. The uterus is adapting to a thinner lining because the body is adapting to shifting hormone levels. Bleeding between periods can be minimized by taking the pill according to the directions on the label, which is often every day at the same time.

Nausea

When taking the tablet for the first time, some people report feeling a little queasy, but this normally goes away. The pill may aid if taken with food or at night. When it comes to birth control, people shouldn't have to constantly feel ill. Talk to a doctor if the nausea is severe or lasts more than a few months.

Breast tenderness

Taking birth control tablets may cause breast discomfort, particularly in the early phases of usage. Tenderness in the breasts can be lessened by wearing a supportive bra. Breasts can get larger as a result of the hormones found in the pill.

Headaches and migraine

Birth control tablets contain hormones that might cause or worsen headaches or migraines. The female sex hormones estrogen and progesterone may set off migraines. Dosage and kind of medication might have an impact on side effects. Low-dose tablets, for example, are less likely to elicit this symptom than higher-dose ones. When a migraine is brought on by PMS, however, taking the tablet may help alleviate the condition.

Weight gain

Weight gain is frequently listed as a possible side effect of birth control tablets, but this hasn't been shown scientifically. Birth control drugs, in theory, could contribute to an increase in water weight or fluid retention. Fat or muscle mass gains may also occur as a result of these activities. When using the tablet, some people report losing weight. Birth control pills' hormones haven't been studied enough to determine if they cause weight gain or decrease, according to an article in 2017.

Mood changes

Hormones have a significant impact on a person's emotional state. A person's mood can be affected by changes in hormone levels that taking the pill may produce. According to a 2016 study of 1 million Danish women, hormonal contraception may increase the risk of depression. A healthcare provider can be contacted if a person is concerned about mood changes. Changing tablets may help if the symptoms are linked to taking the drug.

Missed periods

Taking birth control pills can result in irregular or no periods at all. For this reason: they contain hormones. The pill can be used to safely skip a period, depending on the type of birth control. Find out more by visiting this website. Pregnancy tests should always be taken whenever a woman has any reason to believe she might be pregnant. Pregnancies can occur, especially if the birth control pill is used incorrectly. Thyroid and hormonal disorders, travel, sickness, and stress can all cause late or missed menstruation.

Decreased libido

Some people's sex desire, or libido, may be affected by taking the pill. Hormonal shifts are to blame. The libido of others may be raised by, for example, reducing any worries about pregnancy and alleviating the symptoms of PMS.

Vaginal discharge

When using the pill, it is possible to have changes in vaginal discharge. It is possible that the amount of vaginal lubrication has increased or decreased or that the nature of the discharge has changed. Lubrication can be helpful if the pill causes vaginal dryness and the user wishes to engage in sexual activity. Changes in color or odor may indicate an infection, but these changes are usually harmless.

Eye changes

Corneal thickening has been linked to hormonal changes brought on by the pill in several studies. It's possible that your contact lenses will no longer fit properly, but this doesn't indicate you're at increased risk of eye disease. If a person's vision or lens tolerance changes while wearing contact lenses, they should consult an ophthalmologist.

Cardiovascular problems

It is possible that taking many drugs increases your risk of cardiovascular events such as heart attack, stroke and blood clots. There are some drugs that are more likely to have adverse effects than others. The best course of action can be recommended by a healthcare practitioner. Anyone with uncontrolled high blood pressure or a family history of cardiovascular disease should consider alternative methods of contraception with a healthcare provider.

Cancer

Some kinds of cancer are influenced by the natural female sex hormones (estrogen and progesterone). In the same way, hormonal methods of birth control can either increase or decrease cancer risk.

Fertility Awareness: What You Should Know

How many times have you been told that a menstrual cycle should last 28 days and that ovulation normally happens on Day 14? This is nothing more than a myth. Sadly, it's so commonplace that it's responsible for a large number of unintended pregnancies. Many couples who wish to become parents are unable to do so because of this. The Rhythm Method, which is now mostly out of date, is responsible for much of this nonsense, which believes that a woman's cycle length, while it may not be exactly 28 days, is reliable over time. In the end, it's just a poor statistical prediction based on the average of previous cycles used to estimate future fertility.

In truth, women's cycles are unique to each individual. Remember that the average cycle length is between 21 and 35 days. As you can see from this anecdote, which some religious clients of mine told me decades ago, the Day 14 myth has the power to profoundly alter individuals' lives.

May 21 was the day that Jolie and Mike tied the knot. As soon as they were married, they knew they wanted to start a family, so they scheduled the start date of their joint medical insurance for May 15. They were delighted to learn during their honeymoon that Jolie was pregnant, given how quickly they'd planned their wedding. After her last period began on April 19, the insurance company refused to cover the pregnancy and delivery, arguing she must have gotten pregnant three weeks before the wedding because her last period began on April 19.

'We were both virgins up until the day of our wedding,' she said. She tried to explain to them that since she started running and dieting in order to become a "picturesque bride," her periods had gotten longer and more irregular.

Insurers wouldn't take well to the idea. A pregnancy wheel, which doctors use to determine a woman's due date, was followed by them. Ovulation is assumed to occur on Day 14 based on this premise. It was over for us," Jolie mourned. In a courtroom, how does one prove one's virginity? Moreover, why should this be anyone else's concern?

Jolie and Mike's lives were ruined by the Day 14 fable, to put it mildly. Because their kid was born three weeks after the insurance company's due date, it was the only thing they could take away from their experience. Ilene said he was "worth all the bother," and he was.

The Fertility Awareness Method is a relatively new and very accurate way of determining a woman's reproductive phase, thanks to breakthroughs in our knowledge of human reproduction (FAM). Simply put, the goal of Fertility Awareness is to increase one's knowledge of human reproduction. If a woman is or is not fertile at a certain period, it may be determined using scientifically validated fertility signals that have been seen and recorded. Cervical fluid, waking temperature, and cervical posture are the three most common fertility indicators (this last one being an additional sign that simply corroborates the first two). Natural birth control and pregnancy attainment can be achieved using FAM, and it is also a fantastic tool for diagnosing and understanding your gynecological health issues.

THE MYSTERY OF THE FERTILITY AWARENESS METHOD (FAM)

FAM's greatest obstacle to recognition has been its affiliation with the Rhythm Method, which is a dubious comparison. Those who are ethically opposed to the use of artificial methods of birth control often employ natural methods of birth control. FAM is sometimes misunderstood by the general public. Many women have been drawn to using FAM since it does not include the hormone-disrupting chemicals found in other techniques, such as the pill. Another benefit is that it reduces the frequency with which people are forced to take preventive measures that are uncomfortable, impractical or lack spontaneity. Other than taking control of their fertility and reproduction, many of these folks have a more natural and health-conscious lifestyle.

Many religious individuals have come to appreciate the advantages of Fertility Awareness, even if they don't strictly follow Natural Family Planning (NFP). In contrast to FAM, those who use NFP abstain rather than use barrier methods of contraception throughout the woman's reproductive phase. FAM and NFP users may disagree on ideals, but the desire for effective natural contraception unites them all.

Absence of FAM in Medical School

Despite this, why isn't FAM more widely known as a form of birth control and a means of getting pregnant? One of the most important and perplexing reasons for its obscurity is the fact that medical students are still rarely exposed to a complete treatment of this scientific method. Incredibly, women who use the Fertility Awareness Method know more about their own fertility than gynecologists, despite the latter's specialized training.

A striking exclusion from medical school curricula is that of Fertility Awareness teaching, whose efficacy is based solely on biological principles. Many hormones, including FSH, estrogen, luteinizing hormone and progesterone, have been scientifically established to play a role in the reproductive process. It's even more surprising that the Fertility Awareness Method isn't part of a thorough medical education because it's effective for more than just birth control and pregnancy.

There are a number of disorders for which FAM can be an invaluable tool for doctors and their patients, including:

- Occurrence of miscarriages
- Insufficient progesterone levels
- Hormonal imbalances (such as polycystic ovarian syndrome, or PCOS)
- Infertile cervical fluid
- Short luteal phases (the phase after ovulation)
- Late ovulation
- Anovulation (lack of ovulation)

The ability to more accurately diagnose gynecological issues is another benefit of keeping track of fertility symptoms. Women who keep a chart are better able to assist their doctor in identifying any irregularities in their cycles since they are more familiar with what is normal for them. Charting your gynecological health on a regular basis might help identify potential issues, such as:

- Miscalculated date of conception
- Premenstrual syndrome
- Breast lumps
- Cervical anomalies
- Urinary tract infections
- Vaginal infections
- Irregular or unusual bleeding

Doctors are missing out on a valuable resource if they aren't trained in FAM counseling techniques. Even more so, this can lead to unneeded, intrusive tests to identify an apparent menstruation condition. If women were taught how to track their fertility-related health, they wouldn't need to see their doctor nearly as frequently, and unnecessary medical treatments may be avoided. Of course,

Charting would indicate a wide range of potential obstacles to pregnancy, as the preceding list should demonstrate, ranging from a woman's failure to ovulate to her failure to produce the cervical fluid required for conception. It's possible that this woman has had multiple miscarriages, but neither she nor her doctor was aware of it. The worry many women have when they run to the store or their physician for pricey and unpleasant pregnancy tests can be eliminated by charting. Women who keep a chart can eliminate the uncertainty of a "late period" by tracking their waking temperatures and determining if they are indeed pregnant.

Politics, Profit, and Natural Contraception

Another reason this type of birth control isn't more widely known or pushed is that it's not profitable for doctors or pharmaceutical firms like those who offer hormonal methods like the pill or IUDs. For those that use FAM, there is no additional expense beyond the purchase of a thermometer and possibly a book, class, or app. It's a bargain compared to the pill, which may run upwards of $600 each year!

Is it any wonder that the medical establishment does not push FAM more enthusiastically, given the profitability of so many alternative contraceptive methods? Fertility Awareness is a strategy of birth control that is frequently misrepresented by pharmaceutical corporations because of the large sums of money they spend promoting the pill as a contraceptive panacea.

A pamphlet entitled "Contraception: The Choice Is Yours" asserts that "Natural Family Planning is based on the fact that fertilization is most likely to occur immediately before, during, and just after ovulation." This is a blatant omission of relevant information. Fertilization cannot take place without an egg present; thus, this would nearly make sense, except for the minor fact that fertilization cannot take place before the egg is released!

Of course, the overall portrayal of FAM and NFP is more important than any particular misstatement. For example, the "Natural Family Planning," "Natural Family Planning," and "The Rhythm Method" headings in this brochure were all the same.

The people and companies offering the high-tech reproductive treatments that have given so many people hope have little motive to promote a virtually free system of knowledge that could eliminate the need for their services aside from birth control.

The "Palatability" Language

As a final note, FAM is underappreciated due to its unfortunate label as "unpalatable" by many, particularly in the media. What's going on here?

Every week, a Seattle television news anchor featured a doctor as the subject of a medical segment. While conceding that he truly believed in the effectiveness of the Fertility Awareness Method, he was always noncommittal when I asked him about producing an article on it. I couldn't understand why he thought it wasn't appropriate for the news until he finally revealed that he thought the subject was simply unappealing to the general public.

Perhaps he was concerned about the word "cervical mucous," which is used to describe one of the three reproductive indications. Perhaps if it were referred to as something less obscene, he would think it appropriate for the nightly news. When I suggested that he use the phrase "cervical fluid" instead, he called me right afterward to say that he thought the adjustment in vocabulary was all that was needed to make FAM suitable for the news. He was right, of course. A few weeks later, he published an article on Fertility Awareness Day.

It was only after going through that ordeal that I realized the importance of language in fostering FAM acceptance. Using the more neutral word "cervical fluid" instead of "cervical mucus" has made people infinitely more attentive and interested in FAM since that news article years ago. Consider that the cervical fluid is equivalent to the seminal fluid in women, which may explain why this nomenclature has become more accepted. Although the seminal fluid is never referred to as seminal mucus, its function in both men and women is the same: to nourish and provide a medium for the sperm to migrate.

It's no secret that the media propagates a sterile, idealized vision of the bodily processes that make us human. Although FAM's primary goal is to educate individuals about their bodies' functioning, its ultimate goal is to empower them. In order to make this process easier, it may be necessary to develop a word like "cervical fluid."

WHY SOME DOCTORS FAMILIAR WITH THE FERTILITY AWARENESS METHOD DO NOT INFORM THEIR PATIENTS

In spite of this, many doctors realize that FAM is a scientifically validated, natural technique of efficient birth control as well as pregnancy attainment and health awareness, but they may cite numerous reasons why they do not offer it to their patients. Some argue that women aren't interested in learning it since it's tough, time-consuming, and demands a high level of intelligence. However, I don't believe these claims are true for the vast majority of women.

FAM is actually quite simple and straightforward once you understand its fundamental ideas. (This book teaches the ideas most people need to know.) Alternatively, you could enroll in a course taught by a licensed instructor who can cover all the material in a few sessions.) Learning to drive a car, for example, follows a similar process. At first, it may seem daunting, but with practice, you will gain the confidence you need.

FAM lectures might be intimidating to some doctors because they assume that women are incapable of grasping or assimilating the material that is presented to them. However, I can understand why they hold this view, which is discouraging to me. It's true that FAM attracts a lot of educated folks. Rather than the innate intelligence necessary to operate technology, I believe this is more a product of how people first learn about it. Until recently, only a select few people had access to information about a subject that required a lot of time and effort to learn about.

I've personally taught FAM to over 1,500 customers and can vouch for the fact that almost all women can quickly and easily comprehend the strategy and its biological basis. Furthermore, I believe that the few minutes a day it takes to fill out the application weighs heavily on the minds of very few of them.

In Defense of Doctors

Nothing in the preceding should be construed as a criticism of the medical establishment. In truth, I believe that the vast majority of doctors are genuinely kind and compassionate individuals who are committed to providing their patients with the information they need to stay well and strong. However, many doctors may be suspicious of FAM since it is so low-tech in an increasingly high-tech sector. In fact, if they don't prescribe medications or do other treatments, they may feel that they aren't doing enough for their patient's well-being. As a result, few women learn the approach because clinicians don't have time to adequately explain it during a routine office visit.

In the end, even doctors who advocate for women to take control of their reproductive health can't be as effective as they would like to be if their patients don't keep track of their medical history. Women's cycles must be charted to make FAM a more prevalent practice in the doctor-patient relationship.

3

A Historical Look At The Female Menstrual Cycle And Birth Control

To say that any discussion about contraception must include one regarding the monthly hormonal cycle of women may seem apparent. Every method of birth control relies on knowing when and how ovulation occurs in order to prevent conception. This is true whether you use a pill or keep track of your temperature.

Despite the fact that we use the term "birth control" and surely hope that the techniques we use would prevent conception, what we are truly managing and altering is the monthly menstrual cycle. In addition to knowing how effectively her strategy works, a woman needs to know how it works over the long and short term. In 10 minutes, your doctor may provide you with figures on efficacy, such as the pill being 99.9% successful. True bodily knowledge is required, however, to have a complete understanding of how and what the pill works.

The cultural beliefs we assimilate about periods and the body metaphors we become familiar with while we are practically children impact our contraceptive decisions to a considerable extent. Most women learn early in life about the physiological processes that lead to menstrual bleeding. In most cases, the knowledge is scientific in nature, and we typically learn it when we are still quite young (somewhere between ages ten and fifteen). For the majority of us, that's the end of it, and we see no need to revisit or complicate the information we acquired in health class in middle school or possibly from a parent.

When it comes to one of the most fundamental female body functions, there has been a remarkable lack of public discussion. Before we get into the reasons for this, let's review what a monthly cycle consists of for those of us who haven't taken health classes in a while. Female babies are born with all the cells necessary to develop into eggs. A man's body, on the other hand, produces fresh sperm all the time. When a woman is born, she already has everything she needs to become a mother. Approximately 450,000 of these cells are thought to be in existence (although, of course, every person is different). Age has an effect on this value.

Periods begin for biological females when they are sexually mature. The hypothalamus, a small gland in the brain, begins a complex chemical reaction that finally results in monthly bleeding when enough hormones are flowing through the body. Menstruation begins "up here" rather than "down there," which is contrary to the common belief among women that the sensations of our body are "all in our thoughts."

Hunger, thirst, libido, and drowsiness are all controlled by the hypothalamus, which is located right above the brain stem. Chemical communication is sent to the pituitary gland, which is a pea-sized protrusion just below the hypothalamus at the base of the brain at some point in time. Follicle-stimulating hormone (FSH) and luteinizing hormone (LH) are produced by the pituitary in collaboration with the hypothalamus, much like a group of coworkers working together on a new project (LH). Initially, the body produces a lot of FSH and not enough LH. Ovarian follicles respond to this hormone in a similar way to seeds to water, prompting numerous to sprout, but only one will develop into a mature egg. The uterine lining thickens as the follicles mature, releasing estrogen as they do so.

Many factors contribute to this thickening, including the chance of pregnancy. Estrogen levels rise, causing a variety of additional effects. Because of the thicker and longer-lasting nature of the cervical fluid (also referred to as cervical mucus), they first modify the cervical fluids (sometimes termed cervical mucus). Secondly, the hypothalamus and pituitary transmit a communication to each other, resulting in the release of a rush of LH.

Several follicles have been maturing and preparing to produce an egg up to this moment. During the LH burst, the ovaries induce one (or occasionally two) follicles to race ahead of the rest to burst, resulting in an egg being produced for unknown reasons. The egg is transported down the fallopian tube by microscopic hair-like projections called cilia, and it has a brief life span of around twenty-four hours. No matter whether the egg has been fertilized or not, the follicle from whence it emerged will continue to function throughout its travels. Because of its continued production of estrogen and mostly progesterone, the burst follicle is now known as a corpus luteum (yellow body). Progesterone has two purposes: to keep a woman from becoming pregnant and to signal the body to stop producing eggs. When you're using the fertility awareness approach (which we'll speak about in more detail later), it tells you when you've ovulated, and it boosts your body temperature.

Atherosclerosis in the lining of the uterus prevents oxygenated blood from reaching the fetus. A woman's menstruation occurs when the blood in the lining pools and gathers until it bursts forth, bringing the uterine lining with it. After a woman has ovulated, she is more likely to experience this.

First and foremost, you'll note in this explanation that the menstrual cycle is quite complicated. Every day of the month, not only the days when we are bleeding, is affected by this complex, multifaceted, and cyclical process. When a woman's hormones are altered, her body's everyday functioning is altered. This is a major consideration in the decision to change a woman's hormone levels.

A year or two after starting their period, many women's attitudes on the procedure have shifted. The thrill wears off when women realize they'll have to deal with monthly periods for the next 40 years or more. It's not just our bodies that make us feel less favorable about menstruation; it's also the way we think about it.

Various cultural discourses vie for our attention from the minute we learn we will menstruate, slightly altering our perspective on the experience. The work of second-wave feminism has unquestionably enhanced the social dialogue surrounding menstruation concerns, but even educated women with access to decent health information have a shocking lack of awareness about how their bodies operate and a reticence to publicly discuss their periods. Menstruation is just the beginning of the silence, which extends to questions of contraception and sexual orientation. To understand our complex relationship with menstruation, let's dig further into its history.

The History of Menstrual Politics

As long as women have had periods, people have been puzzled as to why and what it all signifies. According to Alma Gottlieb and Thomas Buckley in their book, "This seemingly routine biological occurrence has been subject to enormous symbolic elaboration across a wide range of civilizations." When it came to studying women's anatomy and physiology, the ancient Greeks led the way. When it came to obtaining genuine human organs, they couldn't do it since dissecting corpses wasn't allowed. The Greeks hypothesized that the uterus was a multicompartment appendage with tentacles based on their observations of animal organs and the behavior of live women.

When it came to the topic of whether menstruation was beneficial or harmful to both women and the society around them, the debate began much earlier. A concept of health based on the four "humor," substances in the body that Hippocrates believed must be in balance to avoid sickness, is still accepted by modern medical practitioners through the oath they swear. Menstruation was seen as a blessing because, among other things, it cleansed the body of harmful humor and restored balance. Aristotle, who was born not long after Hippocrates's demise, had the opinion that bleeding was not necessarily beneficial. According to him, the most significant distinction between men and women may be found in the depths of their hearts. This, according to the great thinker, was where blood fermented and energy was released from the body. For Aristotle (and many others after him), the only difference between menstrual blood and semen was that menstrual blood left the body with a lot of activity, whereas semen flowed more passively. Menstrual blood, they said, was tangible proof of women's intellectual and spiritual inferiority since women's souls have less vitality than men's. The menstrual cycle, in other words, served as a bodily reminder that males are the ones who should be in authority.

It was a long way from where we are now to where we were back then. Perceptions of menstruation remained unchanged. First-century geographer and naturalist Pliny the Elder included his observations about menstruation in his classic thirty-seven-volume work Natural History, in which he "describes menstrual blood as a deadly poison, which contaminates and decomposes urine, destroys the fertility of seeds, kills insects," "withers crops, kills flower, rots fruit and blunts knives." The belief that women's bleeding could harm food supplies has been around for a long time and is still prevalent in some cultures today.

Galen, a second-century Roman physician, was inspired by Hippocrates to assume that menstruation had a medicinal effect. He hypothesized that if the bleeding could reduce women's anguish, it could also alleviate men's misery. While men relied on the lancet to help them get rid of "bad blood," women didn't have that luxury. Many people have relied on Galen to treat everything from illness to poor emotions since his work. Despite the fact that the blood was harmful to the body, it was fortunate that it found a route out of the body. This viewpoint was both negative and positive in the way it imagined menstruation.

Medieval knowledge was based on classical conceptions about the male and female bodies. "The uterus in women is like a toilet that stands in the middle of town and to which people go to defecate," wrote the early fourteenth-century tract The Secrets of Women (Secreta Mulierum), which perpetuated many folk beliefs, including the belief that menstruating women could ruin mirrors, and built new metaphors to explain women's supposed dirtiness at "that time of the month." Bleeding was also compared to "illness," "cancer," and "venomous snakes" in other photos. It is argued by Bettina Bildhauer that menstruation was utilized as the main technique of keeping women in their place because of the association of imagery of contamination, sickness, and uncontrollability with ideas of concealment. It has persisted through the ages and is still with us today, the topic of identifying gender differences, which first appeared in classical and medieval thoughts about bleeding. Blood was the starting point, then the uterus, and eventually the ovaries. Hormones, emotions, and health are all part of it now, according to modern science.

Bleeding was viewed in a different light in the 17th and 18th centuries. The 'pathological' perspective of menstruation was a minority opinion among trained physicians by 1600, according to Michael Stolberg. Women and doctors continued to feel that the female body was riddled with toxins, but a rival method, known as the "plethora" model, was rising in favor as a way to purify the female body. There wasn't a shortage of toxic drugs in women's bodies but an abundance of good ones, according to this perspective. A surplus of healthy blood necessitated evacuation just as much as a surplus of noxious blood. Old notions about body impurity and bleeding were explained in the "iatrochemical" concept, which again compared female genitals to "a gutter." Doctors in the eighteenth century began to believe that the main source of the female body's ills was the uterus, rather than the fluids it contained, like toxic blood.

Through the Victorian and Edwardian eras, the uterus was often seen as a symbol of women's fragility and vulnerability in society. Many new ideas concerning women's health developed during this time period and continue to influence the conversation today. The shift in focus, as explained by Julie-Marie Strange, is due to

Medical community, which "used its empirical assertions to proclaim that science had verified, and might even enhance, the laws of nature," coupled with the "growing professionalization" of medicine. Doctors' use of scientific terminology to convey social notions was obfuscated by this shift from older practitioners who based their views on philosophical and even metaphysical issues regarding women's bodies (in this case, the mental inferiority of women and their lack of fitness for public life).

Women's bodies are designed to carry and give birth to offspring, according to one prevalent theory. As a result, men must devote more energy to their reproductive systems than is really necessary. Thus, a woman's "duties" as a female-bodied person are compromised by her choice to devote herself to mental pursuits, which diminishes her ability to propagate humankind. Menstruation "revealed the susceptibility of female mental health" with traits such as "exalted nerve tension" and poor temper, as evidenced by doctors' perceptions of "mental instability." The present debate over menstruation suppression has its roots in this particular historical era.) There were medical periodicals in the twentieth century that claimed that "if women behaved as nature intended, continuous pregnancy and nursing would render menstruation nearly obsolete." According to this interpretation, women's acts are based on their bodies, while men's are based on the ability to think logically and creatively.

At the outset, this was a difficult formulation: doctors said that menstruation was an indicator of miscarriage, but they also claimed that the absence of menstruation was the primary cause of mental illness. Patients' menstrual irregularities were reported in British asylums by the late nineteenth century, and their return to normal was linked to their mental health. Doctor Anne E. Walker says that "regular activities of the uterus and ovaries were thought to be the basis of 'normal' femininity; abnormalities or dysfunction were considered as resulting in mental disorders such as lunacy."

New beginnings were on the horizon as we neared the end of the 20th century. The belief that the uterus was God's foundation for the rest of the female body, as one physician wrote in 1870, was fading. In the early twentieth century, many doctors began to focus on the ovaries as a source of difference between men and women, a change that would eventually lead to hormones. Hysteria should be banned from medical jargon and from people's minds etymologically, as Dr. James Totherick stated in an article published in The Lancet in 1881. When it comes to recent examples, there's no better illustration than a New York Times piece published in 2006 that asked, "Is Hysteria Real?" Yes, according to brain imaging.") Menstruation, the uterus, the ovaries, or hormones—whatever the topic, there is always an element of women's natural functioning that some people refer to as the source of difference and the idea that women are somehow less than males.

Feminists and a more educated female population came up with their own answer to menstruation being viewed as physically and intellectually burdensome as the twentieth century progressed. They disregarded long-held beliefs, such as the idea that menstruation necessitates rest. The Medical Women's Federation, for example, rewrote the language of menstruation to emphasize activity, cleanliness, and self-control, all in an effort to dispel the notion that menstruation was a sign that women were "out of control" and in need of a man to help them manage their periods on their own. In their view, period-related disease and disability were self-fulfilling prophecies for many women, according to the authors. More educational and professional opportunities would open up for young women if they were educated to engage in normal activities and not regard themselves as sick. Women were urged to educate their daughters about menstruation by promoting programs of youth education and encouraging them to tell their daughters "the facts."

Women were discouraged from discussing menstrual problems with their daughters as a result of this approach, as Strange points out. In order to avoid misleading their daughters about the normalcy of bleeding, mothers should keep their painful cramps to themselves. When it came to dealing with menstruation, the new woman was known for her selective snubs and denials. You wouldn't be able to determine if you were menstruation or not if you were able to "pass" as your non-menstruating self, Sharra L. Vostral points out. Being able to convince yourself that you don't have a bleeding problem would eliminate the need to label you as different or impaired. Instead of challenging traditional gender roles, it promoted them by promoting ideals of cleanliness, self-control, and femininity. Feminists in the nineteenth century argued that women's political power could only be gained by maintaining a ladylike quiet about their periods, and they did so by opposing contraception and relying on widely held notions about female "moral superiority."

During this time period, menstrual product companies like Kimberly-Clark (the makers of Kotex) were claiming authority to enforce cultural standards on menstruation etiquette by building and growing their companies. Pad makers successfully exploited both the feminist vocabulary of liberation and the sexist fears of early century campaigners about self-control and dirtiness for marketing items initially created to bandage war wounds. Until the 1940s, parents were the primary source of information for young girls about menstruation. In spite of the fact that periods were wrapped in a pink mist of secrecy, there was a general societal consensus that if maturing girls were to be protected from the perils of their burgeoning sexuality, it would be by providing them with sufficient information about their bodies. 'Warnings,' she adds, "were used to persuade middle-class parents that teaching their daughters the facts of life was essential in order to keep them from sexual experimentation. To this day, similar diatribes claim that young ladies have too much information at their disposal." Menstruation discussions were set apart from discussions of sexuality, which is a crucial consideration in this context. You talked about bleeding in order to avoid learning about sexual intercourse firsthand.

Respectable middle-class parents debate how to inform their prepubescent daughters of the facts of life in a 1915 guidebook called Almost a Woman. He pushes his wife not to put it off any longer, saying, "I beg of you not to postpone your instruction." Wayne, their father. Right understanding not only protects purity but also develops true modesty," I have come to believe.

If parents were the ones who passed along information about menstruation, there was already a "class of experts" in place. This led to several didactic pamphlets and self-help books preaching on why mothers should teach their daughters about menstruation, as well as why they should tell them in this manner.

The midcentury shift in menstrual authority was seismic as the booming feminine product industry insisted that they, not parents, should be the source of youth education. During the early decades of the twentieth century, tampon and pad makers decided to get into the sexual maturation information industry in a big way, and by the 1950s, they had gained dominance. The big product makers positioned themselves to create and govern the narrative that young girls would get about their bodies by establishing "education departments" that produced brochures and films. Taking on this project had numerous advantages for goods manufacturers. The first benefit was that they were able to establish brand loyalty to their products before any actual bloodshed. It was also possible for businesses to raise the same anxieties that would push women to consume and adhere to their brands by emphasizing the idea that menstruation is something that should be kept private and clean at all times. Some items that promised easy concealment were marketed to girls who had been taught that menstrual management required extraordinary discretion.

As a result, a deep chasm evolved between the upbeat take-home message of initial menstrual education—"periods are normal, and there is nothing wrong with you"—and the lived monthly experience of bleeding—"don't talk about and don't let anyone know that it is happening." As

"To a young girl, if nobody talks about something like menstruation or sex in the actual world, and yet she thinks about it, she's convinced she's abnormal," says Karen Houppert. A woman's period can come with a "one-two punch" of annoyance and create shame, and she says that "women may be thrilled about having their period before it arrives."

It wasn't until the twentieth century that old menstrual myths were given new life in the language of science by new ideas and enterprises. Almost a century ago, Bela Schick proposed that "menotoxins" might lurk in otherwise benign bodily fluids. A plethora of constraints on menstruation behavior may be explained if this were true; perhaps the blood could destroy plants or poison food. According to Buckley and Gottlieb, despite the fact that some scientists still believe in this idea, it was and is "controversial at best." The fear that menstruation blood is chemically harmful persists among a tiny group of doctors and gynecologists. Menotoxins, according to Brazilian gynecologist Dr. Nelson Soucasaux, are actually biological compounds, including prostaglandins (lipid compounds associated with muscle contraction and inflammation response), that are responsible for, among other things, PMS and menstrual discomfort, as well as other symptoms of menopause.

The cultural relevance of menstrual blood can be better understood if we consider the continuation of the concept that menstrual blood is filthy or even harmful. Anthropologist, Mary Douglas, wrote a seminal book in the 1960s titled Purity and Danger, which has had a lasting impact. "Matter that is not where it should be" is how she memorably characterized pollution. In a literal sense, menstruation blood has been viewed this way. Unless we are injured, we tend to conceive of blood as a fluid that is contained within our bodies. Instead, the body's confinement is left undamaged, a phenomenon that has no counterpart in the male genitalia.

A deeper fundamental fear of difference is expressed, according to Sophie Laws, when people worry about their periods being unclean. "The idea that persons with specific features are dirty is very commonly found as part of the attitudes of a dominating group towards an inferior one," she says. Racism and anti-Semitism, as well as misogyny, have a long history of this. She explains that dirt is equated with a lack of self-control, which always has the potential to threaten existing social relationships. Women show cultural "conformity" by keeping themselves tidy.

Inga Muscio's writing depicts a striking image of resistance to cleanliness. A humorous, angry love letter to the female body, Cunt: *A Declaration of Independence*, depicts vividly how the author attempts to both restrict and manage her menstrual flow. On mornings I stroll around with my Blood towel slung tightly around me. When I sit down, stuff begins to flow. It's what I use to clean the insides of my thighs. Otherwise, my feet and the floor will be covered in blood. I get it all over my body when I tread on it. I'm not always quick to tidy up after myself. It's a mess, man. In kindergarten, finger paints can be messy. This is something I enjoy doing for one very good reason: I can!"

Muscio's goal is in part to upset the established structures of female authority that are centered on the menstrual cycle. Allowing one's blood to flow freely is a way of non-compliance. As a queer response to heteronormitivity, her book is lyrical in its reconfiguration of menstruation meanings and gives a clear rebuttal. Despite the fact that most of us wouldn't be happy going about in bloody clothes, it's worthwhile to think about how even the most confident and independent women strive to keep their bleeding a secret and how this concealment erodes their authority and self-worth.

Twentieth-Century Legacies

Doctors have long been seen to be a sign of health when they are absent. Today, we see medical involvement in bodily processes as a proactive insurance policy for better health. Statins and bisphosphonates are used to reduce cholesterol and strengthen bones. Nutritional supplements and medications are available to treat mood disorders. From menstruation to childbirth and, of course, menopause, women's sexual and reproductive health has been managed medically since the turn of the twentieth century.

The women's health movement, which criticized gynecological procedures and pharmaceutical interventions like HRT and the Pill, has had a significant impact on the ebb and flow of this trend. Medical and pharmaceutical intervention, on the other hand, is under increasing pressure today more than ever before. Some doctors have claimed that it is evolutionarily more "natural" for women not to menstruate, but it is up to women to determine whether or not the hazards of HT and ET outweigh the benefits of going through menopause naturally.

Since women's biological processes have been equated with illness by both the medical and pharmaceutical communities, women have been more than willing to take the pills or undergo testing or treatments. Throughout the history of medical writing, this has been a common practice. At times, women's complaints of pain or discomfort were associated with mental illness, and they were frequently advised that it was mainly (if not entirely) their own fault. Even if their mental condition was caused by their ovaries or hormones, it was still mental. While this method was common in the late twentieth and early twentieth centuries, doctors now believe that all discomfort is real and indicative of illness and is therefore ripe for medication or surgery. Both of these methods reveal a glaring lack of room for compromise.

By calling attention to how healthy female bodies were "medicalized" by a medical establishment still dominated by men in the 1970s, women's health activists raised awareness of the ways healthy female bodies were misinterpreted as symptoms of illness. As a result of this new perspective, many women avoided the dangers of poorly vetted medications and unneeded procedures. As a result, women who were coping with true physical pain and suffering were left with no recourse or sympathy. "Buck up, pull up your socks, and get over it" seemed to be the feminist message to these ladies. For the anti-medicalization camp, there were drug-makers and doctors who were more than happy to offer a sympathetic ear to individuals who felt neglected or insulted. They were correct to recognize women's distress, but they were wrong to profit from it by providing unproven medications and pointless medical treatments.

There seems to be an insistence that female symptoms are either totally physical or purely societal, which is the root of the problem. Body and mind are viewed as distinct entities rather than one whole. For the study of culture, psychology and anthropology are the finest options. A person's body is a subject of study in science and medicine. That's a problem because it doesn't account for how culture (including medical and pharmaceutical cultures) can cause illness and how parts of one's body might influence one's identity. A universe in which science and medicine can claim absolute truth is created by this method.

"Until recently, the individual body has been viewed as a universal biological substrate upon which culture plays its limitless diversity," anthropologist Margaret Lock argues. Body differences can only be explained as a result of cultural factors. Medical professionals and proponents of women's health were at odds in this environment. A feminist critique of this juxtaposition is that if medical language insists on being flawless and entirely objective, it implies by extension that activist arguments are founded on subjective, unscientific, and emotional rationales. This is problematic.

In the 1980s and 1990s, this clear and fast separation began to be questioned more frequently. A group of feminist anthropologists tried to highlight the fluidity between many domains of knowledge about human beings and bodies. These new scholars rejected a traditional binary view of the body and argued for "bio-cultural" methods, which meant a way of interpreting physical events (such as menstruation) that included both social and biological components.

A major figure in this process of reinvention, Lock was a scholar and a feminist. After dissecting and recreating arguments regarding medicalization, Lock points out how previously thought-of dichotomies—such as mind/body and nature/culture—are actually interwoven. 'Social classifications are actually engraved on and into the body,' she argues in her essay. Illness and suffering are real, but they are the result of a complicated conversation between physical sensations and the tools our cultures and society give us to evaluate them. Our perception of pain is more important than the actual pain itself. Though you live in a society that views obesity as a symptom of disease, even if you are physically healthy, you may not feel well. When it comes to defining illness, medicalization has been a great achievement because it has been able to hide the influence of social forces.

CULTURES OF MENSTRUATION

To better understand how menstruation has been used to perpetuate gender inequality over the last three decades, feminists have undertaken an extensive research effort. As a result of this cross-disciplinary effort, women have gained a new awareness of their bodies and well-being. As early feminists maintained that menstruation had been misunderstood and unfairly stigmatized, this was an easier task to accomplish. Others claimed that our "poor attitude" regarding menstruation was a cultural aberration and that women who were not exposed to these negative influences would naturally use bleeding as a source of spirituality and empowerment.

This argument has evolved over the past few decades, ranging from being nuanced to being rejected outright. When we understand these shifts and the way we view periods now, we may begin to raise wider concerns about our sexuality, social roles, and ultimately, birth control.

Menstruation is a taboo topic for most women. Women don't talk about it. It's commonly understood to imply "forbidden" or "prohibited," but in anthropology, the phrase really refers to regulations that are sanctioned by a higher power. Until recently, religion held the final word when it came to dictating what individuals and bodies should and should not be like. Taboo is commonly used to refer to numerous cultural customs that restrict or regulate female conduct over the course of her menstrual period. Countless fields of research exist in this area, ranging from African tribal laws prohibiting women from visiting the forest to societies in which women are confined to a communal hut for the duration of their menses to Jewish purity regulations.

For a long time, these restrictions on women's bodies were viewed as sexist encroachments by men. Because males were terrified of women and the blood they shed, they imposed restrictions on the behavior of women during menstruation. "The possibility should not be ruled out that women themselves may have been responsible for the birth of the custom in many societies," argue Thomas Buckley and Alma Gottlieb in a new book on menstrual rituals, which questions more standard conceptions of power relations. The practice of such seclusion may also be voluntary, a cultural choice made by women in their own self-interest rather than in the interests of men when it is carried out. When viewed in this light, women are no longer the victims of societal norms but active participants in them.

People who live in cultures where bleeding women are seen as a hazard to crops can take advantage of this belief by taking a few days off from work. Although it relies on people's unfavorable perceptions about women's bodies, this type of power still grants some degree of autonomy to the group that it seeks to govern. Such a case would be a teen girl seeking contraceptive pills in today's environment. She may be hesitant to tell her parents or a doctor about her desire to have sex, but she has other options.

There's no harm in using terminology that medicalizes her period, such as claiming that her cramps are unbearable. Rather than striving to create new structures and ideas, this is a very limited approach to obtaining control over one's own life.

Menstrual beliefs can be broken down into two categories: those who believe that bleeding women pose a threat to their communities and those who believe that they pose a threat to themselves. A woman's menstrual cycle can place her in a position of strength or weakness, depending on the situation. Medical approaches to menstruation tend to be framed in terms of the former, whereas American cultural discussions of menstruation tend to be framed in terms of the latter.

Premenstrual Syndrome (PMS) is a place where these two approaches of feminine authority come together. According to misconceptions, women with PMS are dangerous or at least inconvenient to others because they frequently express their anger at their partners and coworkers, feel empowered to take time off from work, and indulge in "unfeminine" conduct such as sex acts. They tend to upend gender norms and social roles in general. When it comes to medical solutions, it's important to recognize that they play on patients' anxieties of "harming" themselves if they don't take medication to regulate their hormonal flux. PMS is known to cause sadness, which can be treated with a variety of medications, including antidepressants and birth control pills.

The evolution of the antidepressant Prozac into the menstruation medication Sarafem is one such example that holds larger implications for all pharmaceutical users. Rather than simply rebranding an aging and well-known drug, this scenario includes the creation of a whole new illness that exclusively affects women.

Antidepressant Prozac's patent was expiring in the late 1990s, and drug company Eli Lilly was on the verge of losing control of the popular medication. Because of this, the medicine may be sold under its chemical name, Fluoxetine, by other corporations for a lower price tag. In order to avoid this major financial setback, the corporation employed some quick thinking. To determine whether or not certain women with certain symptoms during PMS have an illness, Lilly held a roundtable of specialists in 1998. Sixteen prominent specialists, FDA officials, and Lilly employees made up the group. The panel came to the conclusion that PMDD, or "Premenstrual Dysphoric Disorder," existed and could be treated with Prozac. To commercialize their medicine for this specific purpose, Lilly received FDA permission in December of 1999.

Rebranding the medicine was unexpected for everyone, even Lilly. They renamed the pill "Sarafem" and launched a campaign to educate women not only about the pill but also about the condition itself. Because they had effectively invented PMDD, women were unaware that they needed to take medicine to treat it. When Prozac went generic and the price plummeted, Sarafem became a lot more expensive while being chemically equivalent.

The events that transpired here raise crucial questions not only concerning the marketing of pharmaceuticals but also about how PMS is seen in various cultures. The fact that PMDD was "created" by Lilly and experts who received funding from that firm does not negate the fact that many women experience debilitating PMS. Women do have more acute and disruptive monthly symptoms; however, this is not the case for all women. As it turns out, the "disease" was created to fit an existing medicine. Pharmaceutical companies developed the societal response to their new health concern by organizing the proper symptoms and giving them a name. Menstruation-related bodily symptoms are a fact; Lilly and its specialists teach women how to recognize, comprehend, and deal with these problems in ways that are both subjective and cultural.

In this case, the border between normal premenstrual symptoms and those severe enough to necessitate pharmaceutical treatment is hazy. It's not like conducting a strep throat test. In the absence of information, it is easy to claim that healthy women might benefit from pharmacological therapy for their monthly hormonal shifts.

In a culture where PMS and menstruation are seen as markers of feminine uniqueness, this suggestion is not out of place. It is culturally accepted that women's bodies are to blame for sexual and gender inequality. The problem isn't a patriarchal social structure that favors men; rather, it's a physiological imbalance that can be corrected with medication.

The author Sophie Laws prefers the idea that periods are governed by etiquette to the idea that they are forbidden in modern Western ways of dealing with periods. Rather than relying on religion or the supernatural, she points out that today's menstruation regulations are based on societal reasons rather than religious ones. Etiquette is defined by her as "rules of behavior governing social relations among people of diverse social positions or classes," and she says that etiquette attempts to sustain established roles by threatening social punishment. Power connections are defined and maintained by this particular kind of behavior.

In terms of bleeding, what are the "rules" of the road that we adhere to? For starters, the procedure is kept under wraps. Menstrual products can be difficult to conceal for women, especially after they've been used. The purpose of this is to look to the outside world as if they do not have menstrual cycles. No blood or gore is ever shown in period product ads; instead, white, clean designs and enigmatic blue liquids are used. Everyday communication is also impacted. Menstruation is a sensitive topic, and it's crucial to know when to start a talk about it. It is acceptable for men to publicly make jokes or other references to the procedure, but it is not acceptable for women to speak about it except in the context of intimate relationships or situations with other people of the same gender. The fact that jokes and statements rife with gender kitsch are the most acceptable context for discussing periods in a co-ed setting is because these forms of speech reinforce traditional ideas about men and women; in other words, they do not threaten established power relationships between the sexes. It's clear that males are still in command, even when it comes to this unquestionably female topic, because they have the authority to start the conversation.

When it comes to women's life, Laws believes that menstruation "highlights an image of women's lives as confined by men's sight." The way men and women connect to each other on this subject, then, serves to remind women that the priorities and aspirations of males are often the ones that govern their life. As a result of this, women who are bleeding are acutely aware of both their own appearance and the males with whom they are in close proximity, as well as the conditions of their interactions with these guys. It becomes more vital to consider how we affect others than how we feel ourselves. According to Laws, "I believe that menstruation is employed in our culture as a fluid and shifting collection of concepts and actions that strengthen men's authority."

Keeping quiet about menstruation in our culture is not only harmful to one's mental health, but it can also be harmful to others. When Karen Houppert, a former Village Voice staff writer, went to buy tampons, she became the first person in the public eye to openly discuss menstruation. A major tampon manufacturer at that time, Tambrands had hiked their prices and decreased the number of tampons in each box by about a fourth, as she discovered.

A two-billion-dollar-a-year giant that holds women globally slave to its whims, the menstrual hygiene industry has become a source of aggravation for Houppert. According to "Embarrassed to Death: The Hidden Dangers of the Tampon Industry," the menstrual product industry is operating relatively unchecked because of culturally enforced silence about all things bloody in the United States.

In order to avoid discussing their periods in public, women were so averse to discussing the issue that important safety risks were overlooked. While Houppert's article's content was obviously contentious, it was the cover that really had people's blood boiling. If you've ever seen a skin cream, perfume, or health club advertisement that featured a woman in profile with her silky thighs and pert butt, you'll recognize this one. But there was a tampon string poking out from between the woman's thighs." Houppert observes that "everybody freaked out," which is understandable. To read the story that was inside, they couldn't even get beyond the cover."

Because of the strong cultural need that menstruation to be kept hidden and private, the response to Houppert's paper served as literal verification of its content: critical concerns affecting the lives of the majority of women could not be discussed.

Breaking the Silence

In my opinion, both the imposed silence surrounding menstruation and the twentieth-century pressure that women feel to pass as non-menstruators have a tremendous impact on their decisions about birth control methods. Hormonal birth control promotes a cultural deception of cost-free contraception in the same way as menstruation concealment does. Only men can benefit from these treatments because of the wide range of health issues and adverse effects that are linked with them. Hormonal contraceptives have the same effect on women's bodies as pads and tampons have on men. Young women learn about birth control while being indoctrinated into appropriate menstrual hygiene.

However, while sex and menstruation are not always linked, they typically share cultural connotations. The topic of adolescent sexuality is one way in which culture, menstruation, and birth control come together. Menarche, or the age at which a woman gets her first period, has declined steadily over the past century, as has been extensively recorded. Many factors could account for this, including a better diet and more exposure to hormones and chemicals in the environment. Tanner's 1976 report on physical development stated that the age of menarche was decreasing by four months every decade. This otherwise unremarkable research coincided with a rising tide of public anxiety over young people's sexuality, leading to a spate of headlines bordering on the hysterical in a number of major periodicals.

Even if a woman's menstrual cycle indicates her ability to conceive, it does not necessarily mean she will engage in sexual activity. In all of these frantic 1970s portrayals of prepubescent girls, menstruation and sex were equated as a metaphor. No one seemed to care that the lack of a period signifies the absence of a pregnancy: early periods meant earlier intercourse and more unplanned teen pregnancies.

In 1991, a Newsweek article titled "The End of Innocence" resurrected the topic of early adolescence. Even though much had changed in American life, the piece was strikingly identical to those written an astonishing 15 years prior. In addition to single and working mothers and famous media villains, the rise of HIV/AIDS was implicated in precocious adolescence. The author's choice of the phrase "breakdown of authority" in describing the impact of both early menstruation and absent parents is telling. The "breakdown" of the uterine lining and the "breakdown" of the conventional family, early bleeding and early sex, and the presence of menstrual blood and a threatened social order are all comparisons that may be derived from this.

Words like "breakdown," according to Emily Martin, are a reflection of how we understand the processes of the female body in the first place. According to her, "unacknowledged cultural sentiments [may] infiltrate into scientific writing through evaluative terms." Menstruation is still portrayed in literature as 'sloughing,' 'dribbling,' 'discharge,' 'shedding,' 'shrinking,' 'deterioration,' and 'disintegration,' according to other authors. Menstruation is often referred to be a sickness by clinicians who choose to describe it in terms of pathology.

For example, the female body is typically characterized as a factory that has failed to execute its duty by employing metaphors. This argues that a woman's primary biological function is to bear children and that every period is a chance lost. Society's definition of a female body's purpose is reflected in this, which is regarded differently based on the body's wealth, race, and age. To characterize their menstruation experiences, women prefer to use ideas of disembodiment and passivity, claiming that they don't "feel like themselves" or are "out of control" and that they don't know what to do about it. We also desire a sense of agency over the course of events. Our health and well-being are harmed by bad events that alter our perceptions of the world. Despite the fact that menstruation can be physically and emotionally painful, it is feasible to claim that the deeply entrenched belief that periods are a sign of our failure to be autonomous and effective may be a contributing factor. There is no truth to that: we are excellent at our work, at managing our lives, and at juggling an astounding number of obligations, duties and responsibilities. We also know that as women, we have to work a little harder to obtain all of this—we constantly have to prove our worth to others. The problem is that many of us believe that we are in control. Monthly, we are reminded that our identities, accomplishments, and ways of relating to others are all constantly mediated by social factors. We aren't free of inequality. We want to show society wrong, to be powerful and accountable only to ourselves, and to be spotless. We want to be free of all responsibility.

When it comes to menstrual management, Laura Kipnis's cultural critique of feminism and femininity, there is a connection between the women's fear of filth and their concern with menstrual hygiene products. Cleaning not only our bodies but also our homes, our faces, and even our relationships makes us feel guilty. Even the little imperfections in our personal and professional lives seem to be crying out for a thorough cleaning. Is it possible that the cleaning imperative would have taken hold a little less successfully if women didn't menstruate? Would it have been abandoned with a little more urgency? Won't the latest miracle cleaning product marketing campaign fail because women don't have a vagina? Would cleaning requirements be relaxed if women didn't have a vagina? instead of only doing half the housework?" As of now, she says, we shall continue to ponder these questions. It's a struggle to keep a house clean in any sense of the word: "Cleaning the house, cleaning society, cleaning up sex."

Sex is where societal cues about cleanliness are strongest. That so many modern women are willing to take on the burden of contraception if it means having sex without the mess of latex and spermicide, as well as the joint accountability, is understandable. It's far more expensive to prevent the possible catastrophes of unrestricted sexual conduct than it is to simply allow it to flow freely. Given this, it's understandable why women might be interested in a medication that claims to regulate both sex and blood.

4

Menstruation And The Menstrual Cycle

ATTITUDES TO MENSTRUATION

Women's periods are the subject of many myths, taboos, misconceptions, and outright lies, all of which can be found in writing, thought or spoken. Menstruating women and menstrual blood's power were formerly thought to be so powerful that they are now considered archaic. We believe that these attitudes have improved. But how much progress have they made?

Pliny's work on menstruation and its effects, written in the second century AD, has had a lasting impact on medical knowledge. To name a few of her supposed superpowers, he held that a woman's menstrual cycle could sour wine, kill bees, dull blades, discolor mirrors, make dogs crazy, and more. I'm sure he wasn't even the very first. Democritus said in the fourth century BC that 'a girl in her first menstruation should be carried three times around the garden beds so that any caterpillars present would suddenly fall and die.'"

Most people thought that menstrual blood was dangerous to anyone near a lady who was having her period, as well as anyone else in the vicinity. Period pain was even supposed to be caused by its toxicity, which produced tissue damage and suffering. Having sex with menstruation women was also a death sentence, either because of the blood itself or because of a Church rule. At the very least, a child produced as a result of such an act would be malformed, leprous, have red hair, or be a female!

When it comes to women, menstruation women, in particular, scholars have written for centuries about the intrinsic fragility and toxicity of the genitals. The male was the benchmark of normalcy, and the female was his inferior 'other half,' and thus proved conclusively that women were weak. These differences can be evident in anatomies, such as in the direction of the male genitals (which are turned outward) and the female genitals (which are turned back inward).

The humoral theory of humoral homeostasis identified body excretions as the way by which an individual maintained a condition of homeostasis and thus explained the genesis of menstrual blood. Women were viewed by Hippocrates and subsequent generations of physicians as being colder and moister than men. The lack of sweating and the growth of hair on the face and body (both signals of increased body heat) meant that women had to menstruate in order to clear their bodies of 'unprofitable blood.' These findings were supposedly backed up by the observation that women who worked hard and were "coarse" were more likely to have lighter periods or not to menstruate at all.

Galen, who lived in the second century AD, proposed a somewhat different view. Menstruation was a way for women to get rid of the excess blood they had made from food; he said because they were weaker than men and couldn't use all of it (excess blood). Foods rich in moisture and fat increase bleeding in women, according to his research.

For whatever reason, malnourished ladies did not menstruate at all, he discovered. Because they believed that menstruation was essential for blood purification, women who weren't menstrual were considered medical emergencies that needed to be addressed as soon as possible. In the Middle Ages, the popular medical manuals were full of cures for "stopped menstruation." As to why this was occurring, there were a number of ideas, such that the blood was either too thick or the uterine muscle was too 'stiff.' Poor food, mental or emotional stress or lack of sleep might all be contributing causes to a lack of menstruation among Medieval women, according to the Medieval Woman's Guide to Health.

For centuries, a lack of menstruation was supposed to have dangerous implications, such as melancholy, suicidal thoughts and insanity or "mother fits," a form of epilepsy (the mother was the word for the uterus). Blood-letting was prescribed as a treatment, which was clearly ineffective when the underlying cause was anemia, as was frequently the case. Even yet, until the turn of the century, menstruation or some type of blood purification was thought vital for a woman's health, leading to the employment of blood-letting and leeches as therapies.

It's hard to think how tough it would be for women going through menopause to deal with all of the myths regarding amenorrhea. She was thought to grow so deadly if she didn't have her monthly loss that she might harm a baby just by staring into the cradle. They were referred to as witches and thought to be capable of incredible acts during menopause.

Menstruation was the subject of bizarre hypotheses for most of the nineteenth century. Despite his belief that women had the freedom to achieve anything they were physically capable of, he argued in 1873 that they should not study. Women's reproductive systems cannot grow normally while they are pursuing academic goals, according to him, because the female body is unable to accomplish two things well at once. This argument was used to prevent women from obtaining higher education.

Today, myths live on. If a woman is menstruating, she may still be barred from visiting a place of worship or a restaurant because she may curdle a sauce or a soufflé by virtue of her presence. Long-term usage of the 'clean' fruit and vegetable only diet was advised in several books on natural remedies in the 1970s and 1980s. Women who adhered to this regimen, according to the authors, were able to stop menstruating after a period of time, which they believed was only essential when a woman's body was in need of cleansing. The (new) hypothesis that menstruation was required to cleanse the body and remove sperm-borne infections was first put out by an American scientist as late as 1993.

A woman's menstrual cycle lasts roughly three years these days, which is about ten times as long as it used to be. It is still possible to study and menstruate, as well as to be safe and healthy on average. Our understanding of menstruation should not be clouded by antiquated ideas about women's innate frailty and filthiness. The fact that our monthly period is a natural biological event means that, despite its minor inconvenience, most of us are content to have it.

THE 'NORMAL' PERIOD

What is a period?

Every month, most women experience a period, which is the shedding of the endometrium (the lining of the uterus). Menstrual blood may appear; however, it is actually a mixture of tissues and secretions from the uterus inside. Mucus from the glandular cells in the endometrium, blood from the capillaries feeding the uterine muscular wall, small amounts of tissue from inside the uterus, and leftovers from structures within the endometrium make up this fluid. During menstruation, all of these components are expelled.

If pregnancy does not occur, menstruation will begin, with the idea that pregnancy is the usual and expected event and that menstruation is the aberrant event. 'If pregnancy fails, menstruation will begin' In contemporary society, many women don't see menstruation as a squandered opportunity to conceive but rather as a relief because they know they aren't pregnant.

NOTE: The term "weeping womb" refers to the fact that menstruation only happens if a woman is not pregnant; hence some male authors refer to it as the "weeping womb." As soon as a woman's menstruation fails to show up, she is likely to drop a tear. When a woman's period comes along, she is usually relieved, and this may be why the expression "woman's friend" is so common.

The 'curse,' 'that time of the month,' 'women's problem,' or the 'monthlies' are all terms that women used throughout this time period to refer to their periods. Perhaps because they've had a more liberal education and are less embarrassed about menstruating, younger women are less likely to use these terminologies to describe their menstrual cycle.

THE MENSTRUAL CYCLE

A woman's menstrual cycle is regular because she produces varying amounts of sex hormones during her whole menstruation years. Normal levels of hormones, known as the "baseline," do not fall below this level, and it is the hormonal fluctuations above this level that cause cyclic variability. When it comes to hormone synthesis and regulation, the hypothalamus, pituitary, and ovaries (also referred to as the hypothalamic-pituitary-ovarian unit or the "hormonal axis") play an important role.

To communicate with one another, the endocrine glands use hormones, and a mechanism known as the "feedback loop" to form a cohesive whole. All three of these hormones are produced by the hypothalamus: GnRH, LH, and FSH, which are recognized by the pituitary; and estrogen and progesterone, which are produced by the ovaries, which are recognized by the hypothalamus. The production of hormones from each of the endocrine glands changes as a result of fluctuations in the production of the hormones from the previous gland in the chain. This is an example of how the feedback loop works.

Either estrogen or progesterone levels are too high or too low for the hypothalamus to respond to. GnRH is released by the hypothalamus as estrogen levels fall during the menstrual cycle. This is an indication of

Initiation of follicular development in the ovary occurs when FSH is released by the pituitary gland. The follicular phase is a term used to describe this part of the menstrual cycle because of the rapid proliferation of follicles during this time. Only one of the tens to twenty embryos that begin to develop will go on to become a mature ovum or egg. At the moment of ovulation, just one developed follicle is left after the others degenerate (a condition known as atresia).

Estrogen is produced in greater quantities when the follicles grow, and this encourages the endometrium to grow or multiply. The 'proliferative phase' gets its name from this part of the menstrual cycle.

During this time of the cycle, the vaginal secretions are also changing. When estrogen levels rise, the vaginal secretions become more acidic and create more glycogen (sugar). Lactic acid is produced when typical vaginal bacteria react with this.

Vaginal acidity lowers infection risk. The 'fertile mucus' that forms around the cervix because of the increased estrogen levels before ovulation is also known as 'egg-white mucus.'

While the ovum is developing in the most mature follicle, estrogen levels continue to rise. GnRH is secreted by the hypothalamus, which in turn triggers a rise in both LH and FSH, which is hypothesized to cause the ovum to be released. FSH and LH levels begin to diminish as ovulation occurs.

The 'luteal phase' occurs after ovulation. The corpus luteum, the remnant of the follicle from which the ovum grew, is the name given to this stage of the cycle. The corpus luteum now secretes increasing amounts of progesterone and, after a brief decrease, rather consistent levels of estrogen under the influence of LH.

After estrogen-induced endometrial development has begun, progesterone stimulates the growth of glandular structures and blood arteries necessary to sustain the growing embryo. The 'secretory phase' of the cycle, which refers to the endometrium's secretory structures, is another name for this part of the cycle.

To keep the corpus luteum functioning normally, an increase in progesterone causes a decrease in the generation of LH. The corpus luteum regresses after about 14 days, perhaps due to the activity of prostaglandins. Endometrium shedding is a result of a decrease in the quantities of hormones released by the corpus luteum, which is essential for its development, health, and maintenance. The hypothalamus releases GnRH when the estrogen level drops to a certain degree, and the cycle begins again.

Counting the days

A woman's period begins on the first day of her menstrual cycle, no matter what. This cycle's premenstrual spotting is not taken into account and is treated as a separate event.) The 'follicular phase' is the time between the first day of your cycle and ovulation. Most people estimate that this phase lasts fourteen days (but varies from woman to woman). The luteal phase begins after ovulation.

The luteal phase, which lasts from the time of ovulation until the start of the following period, lasts on average fourteen days. The normal length of the luteal phase appears to be linked to a healthy corpus luteum. There are two types of ovarian tissue: corpus luteum (Latin for "yellow body") and corpus cavernosum (Latin for "yellow body").

THE RANGE OF 'NORMAL'

Menstrual cycles and periods are difficult to categorize as "normal" because the range is so large, and there are numerous exceptions that match the definition. Periods last three to five days during the 'textbook period,' which is dubbed as such because it can be found in every menstrual cycle textbook. The underlying assumption is that the luteal phase (the period between ovulation and menstruation) and the follicular phase (the period in which the follicle is maturing between the start of the period and ovulation) will both last fourteen days. When describing the menstrual cycle, it is significantly more appropriate to characterize each event as a possible range of times. Regularity of the cycle, duration of the cycle, the length of the period, the severity of the menstrual pain and the color and consistency of the menstrual discharge are the essential aspects.

The regularity of the cycle

To maintain a regular cycle, the timing of ovulation, as well as the amounts of hormones in the body, are critical. Ovulation and hormonal imbalance are intertwined since a failure to ovulate can alter both the hormone levels of estrogen and progesterone (especially progesterone in the second half) and the ovulation process itself.

The follicular phase, when the ovum is maturing in the follicle before ovulation, is the most variable part of the cycle. Some women may ovulate sporadically while they are at the beginning or conclusion of their menstrual cycle. This means that ovulation may take longer for younger women since they may not have established consistent "communication" between ovulation and brain hormones. Stress and change can disrupt the hormonal interaction and disrupt the regularity of the cycle at this age.

Menopausal women may have an irregular menstrual cycle due to fewer ovules and a greater inability of pituitary hormones to promote ovulation. In the years coming up to menopause, stress is more likely to disturb the regularity of the cycle. It is possible for some women to have a luteal phase that is longer or shorter than that stated in textbooks. The luteal phase depends on the corpus luteum's regular formation and functioning for twelve to fourteen days before it breaks down, causing hormone production to stop and menstruation to begin.

Missing a period

If a woman has had unprotected sex, pregnancy is the most common cause of a missing period. Within a few days following conception, you can get a pregnancy test from a pharmacist, supermarket, or doctor. Despite the fact that blood tests can be accurate 10 days following ovum fertilization, most doctors advocate waiting until fourteen days after fertilization to ensure that a false-negative test is not obtained.

A missed period is typically just a hormonal or ovulatory 'hiccough' brought on by stress in women who have never missed a period before. Both pleasurable and painful events can have a significant impact on the hormonal axis. It's usual for people to miss periods when they're in stressful situations, such as when they're on vacation, when they're going through a divorce or when they're going through a difficult moment in their life.

Unless the woman is so concerned about the changes in her cycle that she exacerbates the hormone balance by becoming even more stressed, a missing period due to stress is rarely a major problem, and the cycle will normally reestablish a normal pattern after the incident is through. When traveling, and even for a period of time afterward, many women have a complete cessation of menstruation. 'Pleasurable' stress can play a role in this, but the quick weight loss caused by illness, poor nutrition, or the inconsistent sleep and activity patterns typical to travelers could be the true culprits here as well. In the event that a woman intends to travel for a long period of time, she should be aware of the risks connected with not having a period, including the loss of bone density.

It's common for women to assume that they are infertile because they have irregular periods, but this is not always the case. If a woman hasn't utilized contraception, she can ovulate at any time and become pregnant. If a woman hasn't had her period in months, she won't know she's pregnant for a while because she won't be anticipating one. Alternatively, she may have done something to endanger the development of an embryo when she finds out she's pregnant after it's too late for a safe abortion.

There are several methods of birth control mentioned in the following chapters if you plan on engaging in sexual activity but do not want to become pregnant as a result.

The length of the cycle

21 to 35 days is the typical menstrual period. It's important to keep in mind that this is only a generalization; some women will

have cycles that are consistently longer or shorter than this. The duration of a woman's menstrual cycle may not be of concern to doctors if she does not have a major medical condition.

It's fairly uncommon for herbalists to check for more subtle indicators of illness, such as a lack of energy or a sluggish digestive system. In some cases, they may include signs of stress and inadequate nutrition, as well as aberrant body weight to height ratio. As long as there are no indicators of illness, the lady is exhibiting her own typical cycle, regardless of how long or short, it is.

Abnormally short or protracted cycles can have negative health effects. Having unpredictable ovulation and bleeding in the middle of your cycle is a sign that you may have a miscarriage. A prolonged menstrual cycle can be a deterrent to a woman's ability to conceive. Certain women are more likely than others to suffer from erratic menstrual cycles. An irregular ovulation cycle is usually to blame; however, this isn't always the case.

Symptoms of illness, such as abnormally short or long cycles, as well as any deviations from the normal rhythm of a woman's own cycle, all call for a visit to the doctor.

The duration of a period

Generally speaking, a regular cycle lasts three to five days. Thyroid issues, anemia, and low body weight are all possible causes of periods lasting less than a week. Longer periods may be a symptom of hormonal imbalance, in particular a failure to ovulate, as progesterone generally helps to reduce excessive bleeding because of its effect on the uterine lining. Systemic diseases and some gynecological conditions might potentially be signs of exceptionally extended cycles.

Those days of pre-or post-menstrual spotting are not counted toward the period's length. Premenstrual bleeding should always be reported because it may be indicative of gynecological issues and therefore warrant further investigation.

The volume of the flow

Normal menstrual loss is 50 ml, and an excessive period is 80 ml or more, but no one measures menstrual loss, and doctors don't either; thus, these numbers are largely useless. Speaking in terms of the necessity of altering sanitary protection is much more straightforward. Menstrual loss is more symptomatic of a woman's desire to change than of her actual need to do so.

A woman's self-assessed menstrual loss is viewed with skepticism by many practitioners. Menstrual blood volume was found to be significantly different among women who claimed to have an excessive menstrual loss in a vast number of big studies. Some women thought they were bleeding significantly when they lost 10 ml, while others thought their periods were normal when they lost more than 300 ml.

PAIN DURING THE PERIOD

Even if it is common for women to experience discomfort during their periods, it is certainly not desired or natural. It's typical, and you'll simply have to put up with it, or 'it's part of being a woman.' Be wary of these kinds of statements. No degree of pain is genuinely normal, as the pain response is a survival strategy signaling that something has gone wrong.

In most cases, ovulation occurs just once a month, and the pain normally begins two years after the period has begun—that is, when ovulation has become regular. Because ovulation didn't occur in that cycle, it's possible for a period to be completely painless.

Reducing stress, along with a good diet and regular exercise, may all help ease the discomfort or pain associated with menstruation. Changing your lifestyle can also help with more severe, crampy pain. While this may appear more serious, it may be connected to aberrant uterine muscle cramping produced by a prostaglandins imbalance rather than a gynecological condition. Primary dysmenorrhea is the medical term for this condition.

Prior to bleeding, any severe discomfort, pain that is located on one side of the body, or pain that is not directly linked with the period should be investigated. However, any discomfort that is bothersome or interferes with one's daily routine should be investigated and treated. "Grin and bear it" doesn't apply here.

Heavy loss without pain

Failure to ovulate is the most common cause of a painless period with substantial loss (where pain has previously been a regular aspect of a period). Although it can occur at any time, it is most common after menopause. A lack of uterine tone is thought to be the root cause of the heavy bleeding, and herbalists treat this by administering herbs to strengthen the uterine muscle and mucous membranes.

Heavy loss with pain

For centuries, menstruation was viewed as a noxious waste product that could inflict discomfort just by touching the body. Diets to purify the body, minimize blood toxicity, and alleviate pain were frequently recommended as therapies. Recommendations like these are often successful since changing one's diet can affect prostaglandin levels, which are responsible for pain.

We now know that estrogens and/or prostaglandins imbalance and/or overstimulation of the uterine lining can both cause significant loss and pain. Treating the 'Liver' to improve estrogen excretion and changing the diet to adjust the prostaglandins ratio are common herbal treatments for these symptoms.

Very slight loss with strong crampy pain

The imbalance of prostaglandins and uterine muscular spasms are linked to these symptoms. Natural therapists see these symptoms as a sign that the uterine muscle needs to be calmed and relaxed, but they may also suggest a general need for calming and soothing remedies during the menstrual cycle, as well. For these symptoms, a spasmolytic and nerviness are recommended.

COLOR AND CONSISTENCY OF MENSTRUAL LOSS

The type of menstruation loss is essential to natural therapists because it can be used as a diagnostic tool and an indication of the type of remedy, or even the specific remedy, to administer. Due to a lack of precedent in medicine, medical practitioners are less concerned about determining exactly what is going on with menstruation loss.

Both systems are based on completely distinct systems and require various kinds of information to assist in prescribing. This does not make one or the other approach better or more thorough. As a collection of correlations, the following does not constitute a diagnostic system in its own right. At least two other symptoms of the disease must be present in order for these signs to be considered pathological.

Bright red blood

As a general rule, bright blood indicates a healthy menstrual cycle; nevertheless, bright and flaming blood was previously more common when there was too much heat. For example, an infection in the pelvic organs or a tendency to be 'Hot' or 'Choleric' may be to blame. 'Cooling' herbs or astringents may be needed if the blood is bright red.

Dark, brown or thick blood

Menstrual flow sluggishness is suggested to be a factor in dark blood that is overly thick, aged, or brown. It's very common for some ladies to lose a lot of blood in a very dark red color.

This implies that the patient has to be treated with an anti-spasmodic, uterine tonic, emmenagogues, or a spasmolytic to assist the uterine muscle in relaxing.

Watery, thin or pale blood

It is important to note that pale pink blood suggests poor blood quality and may signal a need for blood-enhancing medicines or hormone management. When a woman is weak, weary, overworked, or undernourished, her hormones may be out of whack, resulting in pale menstruation. Abnormally heavy menstrual bleeding is not uncommon following uterine surgery such as curettes and terminations.

Clots

Most clots occur when the anticlotting elements normally present in menstrual blood cannot retain the blood in a fluid state as a result of the volume lost during menstruation's heavy flow. Clots may suggest that the uterine tone has to be improved by either astringents or emmenagogues.

A PERIOD OUT OF THE ORDINARY

At some point in their menstrual life, nearly all women will experience at least one "weird" period; others will experience numerous "strange" periods. It's possible that the flow is irregular, that the color and consistency have changed, or that the pain is a new or distinct aspect. The essential questions include:

- Is it possible that there is a pregnancy?
- Are there other symptoms of ill-health?
- Has there been a stressful episode (either pleasurable or difficult)?

You should seek medical attention if one of the first two questions is true. Relax and wait for another cycle to see what occurs if the third alternative is a possibility. An irregular period may be delayed if you worry about it.

5

Hormones: Maintaining An Orderly Menstrual Cycle

In a way, maintaining hormonal balance is like staging a multi-act drama in which each of the several hormones has a distinct part in performing. The performers, directors, and managers of the monthly drama known as the menstrual cycle are hormones, the tiny compounds transported in the blood and detectable by blood tests. This play's managers, directors, and players must all work together seamlessly in order for each act to go off without a hitch. Every one of the 'actors' in the hormonal drama is a 'steroid hormone,' as the name implies. Structurally, androgens, estrogens, and progesterone are all related since they all contain cholesterol as a primary building block. The body responds to each hormone in a unique way because of the slight variations in its structure.

The body converts cholesterol into the five primary classes of steroid hormones in response to a range of biochemical and other cues. Pregnenolone (a precursor to progesterone), progesterone, testosterone, and estradiol are all possible outcomes of this process.

It is possible that the hormone at the end of the line will change into a different form, a different type of hormone, or be broken down and ejected from the body as the cycle continues. The 'feedback loop' is responsible for controlling the synthesis of hormones. The brain, pituitary gland, and ovaries form a feedback loop that regulates the number of hormones produced. Hormone levels fluctuate regularly as a result of interactions with other hormones. An increase in one hormone causes the production of its opposite mate to be cut back.

The feedback control kicks in, and the synthesis of the partner hormone is restarted when the level lowers. This sort of feedback loop governs the production of all steroid hormones in the body. Examples include progesterone and estrogen, two of the most important hormones involved in the menstrual cycle (actors). As part of the feedback loop, both hormones have "triggers" (directors).

- Progesterone production is triggered by luteinizing hormone (LH), which stimulates the corpus luteum in the ovary to produce progesterone.
- Estrogen is produced when follicle-stimulating hormone (FSH) stimulates the follicle to produce estrogen. A rise in estrogen shuts off the production of FSH; a fall turns it back on again.

Hormones also have a way of interacting with the cells they are meant to affect. It's done by attaching to receptor sites, which are specific parts of cells that are sensitive to hormones. It is essential that the hormones stay in a state of equilibrium so that the 'menstrual play' may progress without hitches. As a general rule, estrogen levels should be maintained at a level that is in balance with progesterone and testosterone. The estrogen level must fall before ovulation and then rise again for the period to arrive at the proper time.

THE MANAGERS

The hypothalamus, located near the base of the brain, is responsible for the release and inhibition of a wide range of hormones. In the management of the menstrual cycle, GnRH and prolactin-inhibiting hormone (PIH) are the most important manager hormones (PIH, also known as dopamine).

Gonadotrophin-releasing hormone (GnRH)

A variety of hormones and substances in the blood, as well as the neurological system, are sent to the hypothalamus. GnRH pulses are sent to the pituitary gland every 60 to 90 minutes by the hypothalamus, which analyzes all of this information. During the menstrual cycle, GnRH levels rise, suggesting to the pituitary that it is time to enhance FSH and LH production.

Dopamine–prolactin-inhibiting hormone (PIH)

Dopamine is secreted by the hypothalamus in non-lactating women to suppress prolactin production (the hormone responsible for breast milk production). Hypothalamic neurotransmitter dopamine strongly decreases prolactin production. Prolactin levels can rise as a result of a decrease in dopamine and an increase in the hormone prolactin, which can be caused by a variety of substances, including numerous prescription medicines.

THE DIRECTORS

Pituitary gland communications are received in the form of hormones and nerve impulses. Prolactin and FSH, the hormones responsible for regulating ovulation, are produced by the pituitary gland. 'Gonadotrophin' is easier to comprehend if it is broken down into its component parts. "-trophin" means "to stimulate or make grow," and a gonad is the female ovary (or the male testis). The ovarian cells are stimulated or 'directed' by gonadotropin, which is a hormone.

Luteinizing hormone (LH)

During the follicular phase of the cycle, LH levels slowly rise in response to low estrogen levels. Hypothalamus senses low estrogen levels and transmits GnRH signals of increased amplitude to the pituitary gland as a result. Ovulation begins just before the mid-cycle rise in estrogen and LH, as well as an increase in FSH. Ovulation is caused by LH and FSH; although the specific process is unclear, it happens anywhere between 18 and 36 hours following the surge of gonadotrophin.

Both estrogen and progesterone are produced by the ovary as a result of LH. Increases in progesterone during this phase block the pituitary gland's production of LH, so levels remain low until the corpus luteum degenerates and menstruation begins, at which point progesterone levels decline.

Follicle-stimulating hormone (FSH)

When it comes to the follicle that houses the developing egg, the hormone known as "follicle-stimulating hormone" performs precisely what its name says. FSH levels rise throughout the follicular phase of the cycle, causing the growing follicle to produce more estrogen-producing cells.

FSH and estrogen are linked by a feedback loop—the rise in estrogen causes GnRH to be released and an increase in FSH to occur. FSH synthesis is halted a few hours later when estrogen levels are much greater. Because the brain detects a decrease in estrogen levels just before menstruation and then sends GnRH instructions to the pituitary, the pituitary responds by increasing FSH.

Prolactin

In lactation, prolactin is the hormone that stimulates breast development during pregnancy and later increases milk production in response to suckling. Women who are not pregnant often have modest levels of prolactin that increase somewhat at night, under stressful situations, and during the luteal phase of the menstrual cycle.

THE ACTORS

Estrogen, testosterone, and progesterone are all produced by the ovaries and adrenal glands. Initiating tissue changes in the ovary, body changes connected with physical development and endometrial alterations that lead to menstruation, these 'actor' hormones are called.

Estrogen

Estradiol, oestrone, and oestriol are the three primary estrogens. When people talk about estrogen or estrogen levels, they typically imply the combined influence of these three hormones in the body, despite the fact that each one plays a distinct role in the body's functioning. Hormonal and growth-stimulating effects of estrogens are most apparent during puberty when the reproductive system is first stimulated by the hormone. Abdomen, hips, and breast tissue are all affected by them; they also encourage the development of uterine muscle and its surrounding lining (the endometrium). Estrogen has an impact on skin and blood vessel formation and bone strength throughout life.

When estrogen is present, it stimulates cell proliferation, which is one of the essential activities of estrogen. The number of estrogen receptors on individual cells also rises as a result of the hormone's action. As a result, estrogen-rich environments create more cells as well as more estrogen receptors. Estrogen's capacity to boost cell development and the variety of sites it may connect with cells are both expanded.

The lifespan of the estrogens

The ovaries begin secreting active estrogen each month following menstruation (estradiol). Several estradiol molecules are transformed into oestrone, which is subsequently released into the circulation and reaches estrogen-sensitive cells, where it stimulates growth and development. Prior to ovulation, the ovaries produce their highest levels of estrogen, which stays high during the second phase of the menstrual cycle and then drops immediately before menstruation.

The aromatase enzyme converts androgens into oestrone as a second source of estrogen in the body. 'Aromatization' or 'peripheral conversion' are also terms used to describe this process. Hair follicles, skin, brain, bone and bone marrow, muscle, and fatty tissue all undergo aromatization. Most of the calorie-to-energy conversion takes place in the adipose (fat) tissue, which accounts for 10–15% of the total. The aromatization of androgens in fat and muscle is the primary source of estrogen (oestrone) for post-menopausal women.

Prior to menopause, most of the estrogen is produced by the ovaries, but a small proportion of estrogen is always generated by androgens being converted into oestrone. The supplementary estrogen supply that thin pre-menopausal women may be missing can lead to the development of menopausal symptoms, including hot flushes and vaginal dryness. They may no longer be able to ovulate or menstruate.

Enzymatic conversion further divides estradiol into two classes of metabolites. We contain 2-hydroxyoestrone (the "good" estrogen) and 16-hydroxyoestrone (the "bad" estrogen), both of which are considered to have different effects on the body's development and genetic makeup. For women with breast cancer, 16-hydroxyoestrone concentrations were shown to be greater.

It is not possible to create both of these metabolites at the same time. However, the levels of 16-hydroxyoestrone have been observed to rise when pollutants (xeno-estrogens) with an estrogenic activity are present, but the variables that encourage the synthesis of 2-hydroxyoestrone are yet unclear. They're all covered in the following paragraphs.

Each and every source of estrogen has the ability to connect with a target cell, but all will eventually pass via the liver. Ethyl estradiol, for example, is converted in the liver into a less active form and expelled into the digestive tract (via the bile). There is a slew of possibilities once you arrive. Some of the conjugated estrogens are eliminated in this form in the feces, while gut bacteria-produced enzymes known as beta-glucuronidase act on others. Either estrogen will be expelled in the feces, or it will be reabsorbed back into the bloodstream by these enzymes, which are known as "de-conjugated estrogen." Estrogen travels from the intestines to the liver via the entero-hepatic route.

The kidney is the final stop for all of the estrogen in the body before it is transformed into the extremely weak estrogens known as oestriol and excreted in the urine. It's the foundation for certain pregnancy tests, and it may be used to check on the placenta's health while you're expecting. In compared to estradiol and oestrone, oestriol is a relatively weak estrogen that contributes to the estrogen pool, but its actions are more like those of other plant hormones.

The 'estrogen pool.'

Any discussion of estrogen should cover a wide range of other chemicals that have estrogenic effects in addition to the estrogens produced by the body. These include "environmental estrogens," which are taken as meals or as contaminants of foods, like pesticides, and the phytoestrogens produced in plants, which have many beneficial and medicinal properties. The entire estrogen equation must take into account the estrogenic effects of all of these various forms of estrogens.

Any chemical that has the capacity to attach to an estrogen receptor site has an estrogenic action. Any molecule, even a chemical, with a molecular structure comparable to endogenous estrogen can "recognize" and be accepted by estrogen receptors.

The chemical compatibility of an estrogenic substance with a receptor site is one factor that affects the potency of estrogen-like compounds. The estrogenic impact is typically stronger if the drug has a chemical structure that is similar to estrogen and is recognized by the receptor; conversely, if it has a chemical structure that is less compared to estrogen, the estrogenic effect is typically weaker.

Pre- and post-menopausal women may experience distinct effects from phytoestrogens. It is known that they can have both estrogenic and anti-estrogenic effects, even if the exact nature of their activity is still unclear. This finding has been made in both in-vitro and human studies, including women who consume phytoestrogens. Phytoestrogens have a far less estrogen-receptor binding capacity than natural estrogen. However, because of their capacity to bind, they compete with the body's own estrogen for receptor sites, which can stop the stronger estrogens from exerting their typical effects. "Competitive inhibition" is the word used to describe this anti-estrogenic effect.

In line with the anti-estrogenic effects of phytoestrogens in pre-menopausal women, population studies of Japanese women who regularly take phytoestrogens in their diet show a lower incidence of breast and endometrial cancer than Western women.

By consuming foods high in phytoestrogens, post-menopausal women who are somewhat estrogen-deficient can lessen symptoms such as hot flushes. Plant estrogens tend to exhibit an estrogenic impact once a woman is postmenopausal and has very little estrogen, as indicated by their capacity to reduce menopausal symptoms. This is likely because they are the most prevalent estrogen in an estrogen-deficient environment.

Less is known about the "environmental estrogens" (xeno-estrogens). Pesticides like endosulfan, toxaphene, dieldrin, and chlordecone, PCBs found in a variety of products like hydraulic fluid, neon lights, and the pesticides DDT and DDE, nonylphenol released from "soft" plastics and modified polystyrene, and bisphenol-A, a plastic found in the "lacquer" used to coat metal cans for preserved food, are among the many chemical substances that make up this large group of chemicals.

These substances are present at every level of the food chain and tend to build up in fatty tissue. Pesticide consumption rises when diets contain a lot of foods from top-level predators, such as meat from animals that regularly ingest polluted feed or water or flesh from animals that eat smaller animals. Lower amounts of pesticide residue are likely to be present in vegetables that already have them, and organic food also yields fewer vegetables.

Food that has been wrapped or stored in plastic is more likely to get contaminated with these xeno-estrogens, especially if the plastic is flexible (like food wrap) or has been heated. As xeno-estrogens are soluble in fats, this is a particular issue with diets that are heavy in fat. Additionally, Xenoestrogens can be ingested through drinking contaminated water or breathing air tainted by chemicals from industry or the burning of waste.

These compounds' potential effects on health are unknown. DDT levels are higher in fibroid tissue than in normal tissue, and prenatal exposure may affect a fetus's (especially a male fetus') sexual maturation and later fertility. The metabolite of estrogen known as 16-hydroxyoestrone, which has been linked to breast cancer, can be elevated by xeno-estrogens.

But there are conflicting findings from studies on how xeno-estrogens affect women's risk of getting malignancies that depend on estrogen. While some researchers showed no connection between xeno-estrogenic pesticide exposure and adverse effects, others have shown that mixtures of these chemicals may have significant biological effects.

They discovered that whereas xeno-estrogens alone had a minimal biological impact, combinations of these chemicals exhibited effects that were 1000 times more powerful than those of any one molecule. Despite the lack of proof that xeno-estrogens cause cancer, some study suggests they might make breast cancers that already exist more aggressive. Intriguingly, a Danish study found no association between dieldrin exposure and estrogen-dependent breast cancer but a higher risk of breast cancer in women with non-hormone dependent (estrogen receptor-negative) tumors, which remains unexplained.

Organochlorines are a subclass of xeno-estrogens. The health of the baby could be in danger because these compounds are known to build up in fatty breast tissue and are discharged in breast milk. Breastfeeding has been linked to a lower incidence of breast cancer and has been found in some studies to lessen maternal exposure to organochlorines. It is still believed that the advantages of breastfeeding outweigh the hazards, even if lactation is a pathway of organochlorine excretion.

Endogenous estrogens have a life expectancy measured in days, are only biologically active throughout the years of sexual development, and change from month to month with the menstrual cycle. However, Xenoestrogens are a common food chain contaminant.

They are first exposed during fetal development, remain in the body for years, and their levels increase as people age. It's highly possible that not all environmental estrogens' impacts have been discovered.

Progesterone

Because progesterone is the hormonal precursor of several other steroid hormones, including glucocorticoids, estrogen, and testosterone, it is crucial for numerous metabolic processes in addition to menstruation and reproduction. Progesterone is "secretory" in the reproductive organs. It promotes cellular and structural adjustments in organs with progesterone-sensitive tissue, such as the uterus and breast, enabling these tissues to perform secretory tasks. Progesterone in the uterus induces the growth of blood vessels and glandular structures in the endometrium that can create sugars, enabling the endometrium to support an embryo in development. The level of progesterone drops, the endometrial tissue disintegrates, and it is lost during menstruation when fertilization fails, and the corpus luteum degenerates.

Progesterone causes glandular changes in the breast tissue that allow the breast to secrete milk. When progesterone levels are high, androgen levels are low. However, when progesterone production slows or stops, as it does during the postmenopausal years, androgen levels tend to rise. Progesterone also regulates the levels of androgens, which circulate in women at low levels. The alteration in the progesterone to androgen ratio could be to blame for some older women's facial hair growth and scalp hair loss.

Other effects of progesterone include an increase in bone density, an improvement in fat metabolism, a mood-lifting impact, and a natural diuretic effect. Regulating the effects of estrogen in the breast also aids in the prevention of both malignant and benign breast alterations. It also has the same protective and balancing effects on the endometrium.

Progesterone is also a precursor hormone for the synthesis of corticosteroids, which play a variety of crucial biological roles in the body, such as maintaining stable blood sugar levels, reducing inflammation, and increasing resistance to stress.

The lifespan of progesterone

The corpus luteum, or the remaining egg sac in the ovary, is the main source of progesterone. A little quantity is also released by the adrenal glands. Both the ovary and the adrenal gland use cholesterol as the precursor molecule to produce progesterone. Cholesterol is transformed into pregnenolone and ultimately progesterone in a step-by-step process. The progesterone may subsequently be transformed into estradiol, oestrone, testosterone, or cortisone, among other steroid hormones.

In the blood, progesterone interacts with cell receptors before passing through the liver, where it is inactivated and eliminated in the bile and urine.

Androgens

Androgens are the hormones that cause masculinization; they are released by both males and females. Menstrual cycle and reproductive irregularities, as well as male pattern hair growth, voice deepening, and loss of the feminine body features, including a reduction in breast size, can occur when androgen secretion is too high, as in polycystic ovarian syndrome.

The most prevalent androgen in the blood of healthy women is testosterone. It also has the most power. 25% of the overall volume comes from the ovary, 25% from the adrenal gland, and 50% is created by the conversion of other ovarian or adrenal hormones. When testosterone is present in muscle, it directly binds to androgen receptors to have anabolic (growth-promoting) effects.

As a woman approaches menopause, androgen production naturally and gradually declines. Women in their forties have testosterone levels that are roughly half those of women in their twenties. After menopause, testosterone levels drop by about 15%, and the adrenal glands are responsible for 50% of the generation of circulating levels. Loss of libido, persistent exhaustion and a lack of well-being are signs of the natural drop of androgens around menopause even while estrogen levels are acceptable. As there is no agreement on the clinical definition, this group of symptoms, known as "androgen deficiency syndrome," continues to be somewhat debatable. Additionally, it is debatable whether blood tests are sensitive enough to detect low levels of testosterone.

The main precursor hormone is androstenedione, which is changed in the liver, fat, and skin before returning to the bloodstream as testosterone. In order to avoid the requirement for high blood levels of androgens that could have negative consequences, conversion is thought to take place in the tissues so that cells that are responsive to androgens have a local supply. Both the ovary and the adrenal gland generate androstenedione, although the amount from each source appears to vary depending on the time of day and ovarian cycle phase.

Dihydrotestosterone (DHT) is created from testosterone and androstenedione, and it is thought that an excess of this hormone has masculinizing effects on women, including male-pattern hair growth, acne, and clitoris hypertrophy. The adrenal gland secretes Dehydroepiandrosterone (DHEA) and DHEA sulfate, with minor amounts also coming from the ovary.

Although their function is unclear and they are less physiologically active than the other androgens, levels of DHEA decrease with aging. In the tissues, some DHEA is converted to testosterone. DHEA sulfate is simple to quantify and offers a trustworthy way to assess aberrant adrenal androgen levels. Moderately androgenic Androstenediol is the hormone that occurs in between the production of DHEA and testosterone. Androstenediol levels in hirsute women are double those in healthy women.

The carrier proteins

The majority of steroid hormones are protein-bound and circulate in plasma (albumins and globulins). It appears that each hormone is transported by a distinct binding globulin or carrier protein. The hormones are less able to interact with target tissues when they are bound to the globulins than when they are 'free' in the plasma. Additionally, they are shielded from deactivation and breakdown.

Sex hormone-binding globulin (SHBG)

Estrogen and an excess of thyroid hormone both stimulate the liver to produce more SHBG, which is a hormone that is generated there. Both androgens and estrogens can attach to it. Production of SHBG is lowered by several circumstances. These include insulin resistance, high levels of testosterone, the use of progestogens, Cushing's syndrome-related glucocorticoid hormone excess, excessive growth hormone (acromegaly), and thyroid hormone deficit. By limiting the amount of "free" estrogen that can interact with target cells, the SHBG level regulates estrogenic action.

Cortisol-binding globulin (CBG)

The protein used to transport cortisol and progesterone is called CBG, also referred to as transcortin. More than 90% of progesterone is linked to CBG, which controls the amount of progesterone that is readily available in a similar manner to how SHBG controls estrogen and androgen levels.

6

Hormonal Balance

In good health, hormones (together with prostaglandins) work in concert to start the reactions that result in a regular menstrual cycle. When hormone levels alter, many gynecological issues can become apparent. When a woman enters menopause, for example, these alterations may be caused by an absolute or "relative" hormone shortage (a hormone may be relatively lower than it ought to be or relatively lower in relation to other hormones). This is one theory for premenstrual syndrome (PMS), where a variety of premenstrual symptoms are thought to be caused by relatively low levels of progesterone in relation to estrogen.

On the other side, hormone levels can be abnormally high, exposed for an excessive amount of time, or present at levels that are excessively high in comparison to other hormones. For instance, it is believed that women who have endometriosis and fibroids have been exposed to excessively high quantities of estrogen. Alternately, situations could develop when progesterone exposure is insufficient compared to estrogen's growth-promoting effects. It is known as "unopposed estrogen."

TOO MUCH OESTROGEN

Prolonged exposure to estrogen

The fact why modern women experience more estrogen effects is primarily due to their increased lifetime period frequency. Menarche (a woman's first period) starts sooner on average, menopause starts later on average, and women have fewer children than in the past.

Contrary to popular belief, estrogen excess is not caused by excessive estrogen production by the ovaries; rather, there is typically an issue with the availability and clearance of estrogen. Premenstrual tension, heavier than usual menstruation, and longer than typical menstrual periods are possible symptoms. Relative estrogen excess has been linked to an increase in the incidence of menorrhagia, endometriosis, fibroids, fibrocystic breast disease, and breast and endometrial cancer.

A single blood test cannot identify estrogen levels that are abnormally high since they are comparative. Researchers test their hypothesis by comparing the blood levels and/or length of estrogen exposure (time when periods started, number of pregnancies, breastfeeding, menopause, etc.) of numerous healthy women with those who have the estrogen-dependent complaint. They make the hypothesis that an imbalance may be the mechanism of disease initiation. Estrogens from the environment are another substance that can enter the body and are now recognized as a major cause of disease.

Unopposed estrogen

Because of its proliferation properties, estrogen encourages the growth of tissues that respond to it, as seen, for instance, in the uterine lining. Progesterone must rise and fall sufficiently to allow for normal shedding during menstruation, which guards against endometrial hyperplasia and cancer. Progesterone deficiency increases the likelihood of endometriosis and fibroids, as well as other estrogen-related diseases. Unopposed estrogen may raise the risk of breast cancer in the breast. Based on the knowledge of the protective properties of progesterone in the endometrium, several hormone replacement treatment (HRT) preparations now contain both estrogen and progesterone.

Poor clearance of estrogen

Because of the way that modern women live, which appears to impair the liver's and bowel's ability to remove estrogen from the body and favors higher circulating levels of available (biologically active) estrogens in the blood, modern women are relatively overexposed to the stimulatory effects of estrogen compared to women of earlier eras.

DIET AND OBESITY INCREASE OESTROGEN LEVELS

Diet

A higher risk of estrogen-dependent illnesses, such as cancer, has been linked to diets high in saturated fat, low in dietary fiber, and high in refined carbohydrates, according to epidemiological studies.

Fat intake

Animal fats that are saturated with saturated fats promote the development of intestinal bacteria that generate the enzyme beta-glucuronidase. Women who consume more fat have much greater blood levels of estrogen than those who follow low-fat diets because this enzyme changes estrogen into a form that can be reabsorbed from the gut. On the other hand, decreasing fat intake raises estrogen clearance, which lowers estrogen levels. High fat intake has been associated with endometriosis, fibroids, excessive menstrual bleeding, benign breast illness, and breast cancer.

Obesity

Being overweight or weighing a few extra pounds is not the same as being obese. Women who are more at risk are severely overweight and have BMIs that are in the highest percentile. By interfering with normal ovulatory function, obesity can alter the menstrual cycle. It is also linked to high estrogen levels. More fatty tissue increases the body's capacity to convert androgens into estrogens, which increases the risk of endometriosis, fibroids, and breast cancer.

Additionally, it has been hypothesized that the kind of obesity may be important. Women who have a high percentage of upper body fat (high waist measurement) typically have higher amounts of free estrogen and lower levels of SHBG.

DIETARY AND LIFESTYLE CHANGES TO REDUCE ESTROGEN LEVELS

Diet

Dietary fiber

Dietary fiber lowers the levels of estrogen in the blood and urine, 9 presumably by affecting an enzyme generated by gut flora (beta-glucuronidase).

The amount of de-conjugated estrogen that can re-enter the bloodstream and the activity of this enzyme are both decreased by a diet low in fat and high in fiber. Because vegetarians typically consume more fiber and fewer lipids in their diets than meat-eaters, they have much lower bacterial enzyme activity than meat-eaters.

The fiber found in whole foods is better than morning cereals that solely include fiber and don't contain any other beneficial elements. Fiber comes in soluble and insoluble forms. The gut's microflora can alter insoluble fiber, but the digestive system cannot break it down. An illustration of insoluble fiber is wheat bran. Water-soluble fiber includes mucilage (found in psyllium husks), pectins (found in the peels and rinds of fruits and vegetables), and lignans (as in linseeds). (The soluble fibers have numerous positive effects; they lower cholesterol, lessen blood sugar spikes after meals, increase bile solubility, and encourage the development of good gut bacteria.) When lignans are transformed by the gut flora into enterolactone and enterodiol, they have estrogenic effects. These weak estrogens may, for example, lower the risk of breast cancer by shielding against the proliferative effects of endogenous estrogens.

Cultured milk products and yogurt

The bacteria in yogurt, Lactobacillus acidophilus, likewise decreases beta-glucuronidase activity11, suggesting that eating yogurt and fermented milk products has a favorable impact on estrogen excretion.

Eating these foods has been linked to a lower incidence of breast cancer, which researchers ascribe to either a decrease in estrogen re-absorption or to other immune-boosting properties of the Lactobacillus bacteria.

Phytoestrogens

Plant estrogens, often known as phytoestrogens, have a variety of impacts on the body's estrogenic activity. Through a process known as "competitive inhibition," they can stop body-produced estrogen from attaching to their receptor sites. They can also make estrogen comparatively unavailable by raising levels of the estrogen's carrier protein, SHBG, which slows down the conversion of androgens to estrogen that typically takes place in fatty tissue. Less estrogen is available to bind to estrogen receptors when more estrogen is bound to SHBG.

The cabbage family

The indoles, which are found in vegetables and herbs from the cabbage family, can speed up the liver's conversion of estrogen into the water-soluble form that can be eliminated in feces. Indoles also appear to compete with estrogen to decrease its effects and slow the development of breast cancer cells. Women with estrogen-dependent conditions can frequently eat vegetables from the cabbage family. All varieties of cabbage, broccoli, brussels sprouts, and radicchio are among them. This family of medicinal plants includes Capsella bursa-pastoris, which is used to treat irregular uterine bleeding.

Protein intake

Protein intakes must be sufficient for the liver to process estrogen. It is advised to consume no more than 60 g of protein daily in the form of cereals, legumes, lean meat, fish, organic poultry, and eggs because excessive protein intake is linked to a number of health issues.

Vitamin B6

It appears that estrogen is influenced by vitamin B6 indirectly. The uterus and breast tissues have been demonstrated to be more susceptible to the estrogen-stimulating effects of vitamin B6 deficiency, and B6-deficient women with breast cancer have a lower survival rate. The fact that vitamin B6 functions like a pharmacological agent and modifies the physiological changes brought on by an excess of estrogen may be the reason for its beneficial benefits.

Alcohol

Alcohol has a variety of complex impacts on the metabolism of estrogen and illnesses connected to estrogen. One drink of beer, wine, or spirits per day has been shown to lower estrogen levels and uterine cancer incidence (especially in overweight women), but it has also been linked to an increased risk of breast cancer. It may be recommended for women with additional breast cancer risk factors to limit their alcohol use. Other women, particularly those at higher risk for cardiovascular disease, may benefit from a modest intake of red wine (one to two standard glasses every second or third day).

Liver clearance of estrogens

Bitter plants or foods (together referred to as "bitters") are used by natural therapists to relieve symptoms associated with "liver congestion." Bitters promote bile production, bile salt dilution, cholesterol clearance, and maybe estrogen clearance. Bitters are calming and are indicated for conditions where there is too much heat, such as irritation, acid reflux, migraines, excessively bright-red menstrual flow, dry stools, and face acne.

Unknown is the precise mechanism through which bitter plants influence the menstrual cycle. It's possible that the higher rate of bile flow that occurs while taking bitter herbs will also speed up the hepatic conversion of estrogen. Their principal mode of action may include changing the bacteria in the bowel. However, as bitter herbs are a huge and diverse group with many different functions, the impacts are probably going to be rather complex. Some of them have known uterine actions that are distinct from any estrogen-clearing effects, so they might work together.

Methionine-rich foods help the liver's process of methylating estrogen, which converts estrogen (estradiol) into a less powerful version (oestriol). Onions, garlic, onions, and other legumes are high in methionine.

Exercise

Exercise aids in the removal of estrogen, and women who exercise frequently report lighter periods.

TOO LITTLE OESTROGEN

When too much estrogen is excreted from the body, too little is recycled through the enterohepatic (entero-bowel, hepatic-liver) circulation, and/or too little of the non-ovarian estrogen is produced in the fat cells, a relative estrogen shortage results. After menopause or in situations when there is a reduced ovarian reserve, such as after chemotherapy, pelvic radiation therapy, surgically removing part of the ovary, or while nursing, a real estrogen deficit arises.

When estrogen levels are excessively low, it can lead to low bone density, poor fertility and libido, irregular periods, premature aging, or excessive dryness and brittleness of tissues, including the vagina, bones, and skin.

FACTORS THAT REDUCE THE AVAILABILITY OF ESTROGEN

Body weight

Having a body mass index that is 15% to 20% below the optimal body mass index can frequently cease menstruation and result in estrogen levels that are abnormally low. Fertility and bone density tend to decline, and the cycle can also become unpredictable.

Diet

Fiber

Consuming excessive amounts of fiber, especially wheat-bran cereals, reduces estrogen levels and raises a woman's risk of getting osteoporosis. This issue does not appear to be brought on by fiber when consumed as whole food.

Vitamin A deficiency

Low activity of the enzyme 3 beta-dehydrogenase, which is essential for the generation of estrogen (estradiol) in the ovary, is caused by vitamin A insufficiency and results in low estrogen. Vitamin A is produced in the body from dietary beta-carotene found in orange, yellow, and green fruits and vegetables. (During pregnancy, vitamin A supplements containing more than 2500 IU per day are not advised.)

Antibiotics

The gut bacteria required to change estrogen into its more active form for recirculation are significantly diminished by antibiotics. Additionally, intestinal bacteria are required for the conversion of some phytoestrogens into their active, estrogenic form, particularly the lignans. Antibiotics may reduce the efficiency of natural estrogens used by women who rely on these sources. Yogurt and cultured milk can gradually help bowel colonies, but it's still best to avoid using antibiotics unless you have a severe illness.

Excessive exercise

Overtraining lowers circulating estrogen levels, which can lead to amenorrhea and inadequate bone density. Additionally, an excessive activity that interferes with pituitary-ovarian function when nutrition or energy intake is insufficient compared to the energy expended results in amenorrhea. Both bone density and the number of circulating estrogens are decreased.

Smoking

Smoking changes the metabolism of estrogen, increasing the production of inactive estrogen. Smoking causes a relative lack of estrogen in women, which contributes to earlier natural menopause and a higher risk of osteoporotic fractures.

Phytoestrogens can reduce low estrogen symptoms

Menopausal women and women with a relative estrogen shortage can greatly benefit from phytoestrogens by reducing their low estrogen symptoms. Reduced hot flashes and estrogenic alterations in the vaginal mucosa are just a couple of the estrogen-like actions that the isoflavones, cholesterol, and lignans can elicit when they bind to the estrogen receptor sites. Numerous significant women's tonic herbs include large concentrations of steroidal and triterpenoid saponins, which also appear to have "estrogenic" and hormone-balancing properties. Cimicifuga racemosa, Trillium erectum, Aletris farinosa, Panax ginseng, and Glycyrrhiza glabra are among the members of this category.

Foods and herbs that contain saponins offer added advantages. They can lower blood cholesterol levels and appear to enhance mineral intake by mildly irritating the gut wall, which facilitates the passage of minerals into the bloodstream. Soy products, lentils, and potatoes with skins are food sources of saponins. Bone density can be increased by phytoestrogens. Researchers have so far discovered benefits from Chinese herbal remedies, soy products, and cholesterol (a phytoestrogen).

Higher dietary isoflavone intake from soy protein has been linked to an increase in bone mineral density in postmenopausal women but not in premenopausal women, according to more recent research. In one tiny study, PromensilTM, a supplement containing isoflavones from Trifolium pratense, showed a significant improvement in bone density. Initial studies on the ability of ipriflavone, a synthetic isoflavone, to stop bone loss in postmenopausal women were likewise encouraging. Early investigations revealed favorable results, presumably as a result of higher rates of bone production. Later studies, however, revealed that ipriflavone did not stop the acute bone loss that occurred right after oophorectomy, and in another trial, a sizable proportion of women experienced lymphocytopenia.

Diverse studies have been conducted on the efficacy of supplements containing concentrated isoflavones. A later study comparing PromensilTM to placebo also found that the treatment group experienced a 44 percent reduction in hot flushes. However, a placebo-controlled clinical trial using concentrated isoflavone supplements made from red clover (PromensilTM) did not show any significant improvement in menopausal flushing compared to placebo.

PROGESTERONE DEFICIENCY SYNDROMES

The mature ovarian follicle's corpus luteum, which has matured since ovulation, is where the ovary gets its progesterone after that. As a necessary step in the production of progesterone, this structure is filled with blood that contains cholesterol. If pregnancy develops, the corpus luteum continues to produce progesterone for around seven weeks. If pregnancy does not develop, the period starts fourteen days following ovulation when the corpus luteum dies. When ovulation does not occur, such as with childbirth, miscarriage, terminations, discontinuing the Pill, and when breastfeeding, no progesterone is created. Progesterone deficiency brought on by ovulatory failure is also evident in irregular bleeding patterns, during stressful situations, during and after menopause, and at menarche.

The association between progesterone and gynecological symptoms such as premenstrual syndrome, dysfunctional bleeding patterns, cyclic breast disorders, infertility, endometriosis, and fibroids has been the subject of several studies over the years. Progesterone deficiency is believed to be involved with several illnesses at least some of the time, though there is no universal agreement on this. Progesterone synthesis or availability difficulties, aberrant progesterone levels in relation to other hormone levels, or tissues lacking proper progesterone receptivity are all potential causes of concern.

A number of disorders linked to insufficient progesterone, commonly known as corpus luteum insufficiency, are described in the scientific literature. These include latent hyperprolactinemia, which may contribute to infertility, PMS, and cyclic breast pain, luteal phase abnormalities that produce observable endometrial problems and infertility, and aberrant tissue receptivity that may cause issues with any progesterone-sensitive tissues.

Luteal phase defects

The phrase "luteal phase defect" refers to the endometrium's insufficient transformation during the secretory (luteal phase) of the cycle, which can result in infertility. According to estimates, 3–4% of women with unexplained infertility and up to 63% of women who consistently miscarry are affected by luteal phase abnormalities. Additionally, it has been demonstrated that 6–10% of fertile women have an insufficient luteal phase.

Progesterone insufficiency or normal levels of progesterone that do not effectively stimulate the endometrium have been linked to a number of issues, including:

Abnormal follicular development

The anterior pituitary gland's inadequate release of FSH and LH might result in aberrant follicular development. The granulose cells of the growing follicle are normally stimulated by FSH to create estradiol from androstenedione. Reduced FSH production leads to irregular follicle development, lower estradiol levels, and reduced progesterone synthesis.

Abnormal luteinization

Theca cells of a growing follicle are often stimulated by LH to generate androstenedione. Androstenedione can drop due to an adequate LH release, which can also contribute to the insufficient hormone production mentioned above (a decrease in estradiol and lower progesterone levels). Additionally, a subpar LH surge at ovulation results in insufficient luteinization of the granulosa cells, which in turn results in a lack of progesterone.

Luteinized unruptured follicle syndrome

Failure of the main follicle to release its ovum within 48 hours following the LH blood peak is known as luteinized unruptured follicle syndrome. This is accompanied by reduced estrogen and progesterone levels during the luteal phase. Hormone levels are normal before the anticipated ovulation, indicating that the luteinized unruptured follicular syndrome problem lies within the follicle itself. This syndrome is linked to infertility and may be more prevalent in endometriosis-affected women.

Abnormally low cholesterol levels

All steroid hormones are produced using cholesterol as a crucial precursor. Low to nonexistent progesterone synthesis and luteal-phase abnormalities are brought on by abnormally low cholesterol levels.

Latent hyperprolactinemia

Dopamine inhibits anterior pituitary prolactin secretion while thyroxin-releasing hormone (TRH) produced from the brain stimulates it. When an increased prolactin release is seen after receiving a TRH injection intravenously, latent hyperprolactinemia has been identified. Low progesterone production and an irregular menstrual cycle with a shortened luteal phase have been linked to slightly higher prolactin levels. In terms of medicine, latent hyperprolactinemia is suspected when women complain of infertility, PMS, or premenstrual breast pain.

UTERINE ABNORMALITIES

Even when progesterone levels are normal, uterine anomalies alter the endometrium's blood flow and blood vessel growth. The inadequate development of the endometrium is brought on by fibroids, uterine septa, and endometritis.

Abnormal tissue responsiveness to progesterone

The hypothesis that tissues can lack the typical responsiveness to a spectrum of hormones that generally play a role in the development or function of those tissues is another way to explain how problems with progesterone can occur. The endometrium, the developing follicle, or other progesterone-sensitive tissues like the breast may all exhibit this lack of receptivity. Progesterone production may be aberrant due to tissues' lack of receptivity to progesterone or, alternatively, due to their lack of hormonal sensitivity to FSH, LH, or prolactin.

Lower amounts of progesterone, for instance, will occur when the corpus luteum fails to grow as a result of the follicular tissue's abnormal lack of reactivity to either FSH or LH. Alternately, progesterone receptor binding in the endometrium may be flawed, leading to a delay in the development of this tissue and issues with either fertility or the uterine lining's ability to function during menstruation. Cyclical breast discomfort may be brought on by a shortage of progesterone receptivity in other tissues, such as the breast. The progesterone receptor's diminished responsiveness has also been linked to PMS.

Progesterone and menopause

Ovulation and corpus luteum development is necessary for progesterone synthesis. Ovulation rates start to drop during the perimenopausal years and eventually stop with the beginning of menopause. All women experience a reduction in estrogen levels throughout the month as a result of this natural biological process, which also causes a decrease in progesterone levels during the luteal phase of ovulatory cycles. Progesterone levels are very low in cycles where ovulation entirely fails.

With HRT, attempts have been made throughout the years to postpone both this biological certainty and the symptoms that go along with it. If a woman has a uterus, she is typically prescribed some sort of estrogen with progesterone; if she has had a hysterectomy, she is typically prescribed estrogen alone. Those who adhere to Dr. John Lee's advice are now advocating progesterone as the new type of HRT for menopausal symptoms (marketed as natural or bio-identical progesterone).

Some women have enthusiastically embraced this type of HRT under the assumption that "natural" equates to "safe" or that the absence of side effects equates to zero risk. It may turn out that "natural progesterone" is one of those naturally occurring substances that is actually highly dangerous. Additionally, the absence of short-term side effects is not a reliable indicator of a decreased risk of disease with continued treatment.

MAKING A DIAGNOSIS

Tests or clinical examinations can be used to diagnose progesterone insufficiency. These include keeping a simple menstruation diary, measuring the basal body temperature, figuring out how long the luteal phase lasts, and, for infertile women, progesterone blood tests and/or endometrial biopsies.

In order to determine the kind, degree, and timing of symptoms, a menstrual symptom questionnaire can be completed every day for one or more months. Tension, irritability, anxiety, and other mood changes are signs of a progesterone shortage or lack of availability, which only happens during the luteal phase of the cycle.

The availability of progesterone in the luteal phase can be assessed using basal body temperature, which is measured orally. When the body is at rest, the temperature is taken in the early morning before any activity (including chatting or turning over in bed). The most accurate thermometer is an old-fashioned mercury thermometer. Progesterone has been demonstrated to cause a minor but noticeable increase in body temperature that is 77% reliable.

It is possible to gauge how long the luteal phase lasts. A precise ovulation date is required, and periods that arrive less than eleven days after ovulation are strongly suggestive of luteal phase abnormalities. The basal body temperature, a mid-cycle blood or urine test to look for the mid-cycle increase in LH, or an ultrasound scan to see the growing follicle can all be used to identify ovulation. The most precise method of determining the ovulation date is a scan; the least accurate one is to deduct fourteen days from the start of bleeding.

Progesterone levels in the blood are typically measured seven to nine days after ovulation, and values that are consistently less than 10 nanamol/milliliter are a sign that progesterone levels are excessively low. Progesterone values fluctuate greatly and can go from normal to very low in a short period of time, making blood tests to measure progesterone levels not entirely trustworthy.

If a woman has undiagnosed infertility, an endometrial biopsy may also be advised to assess endometrial development because luteal phase problems are linked to poor endometrial maturation. Since one-third of all women have abnormal endometrial growth, it takes two or more consecutive cycles for the irregularity to be regarded as a cause of infertility.

Treatment

To control ovulation and, consequently, progesterone production, people utilize Vitex agnus-castus, Paeonia lactiflora, and plants containing steroidal or triterpenoid saponins. It is believed that each one of the functions on the hypothalamic-pituitary-ovarian axis is centrally functioning.

Many of the medicinal plants used to treat gynecological symptoms contain a specific class of phytoestrogens called saponins. They resemble steroid hormones in terms of structure. Their exact mechanism of action is uncertain, although they appear to interact with pituitary and hypothalamic receptors to boost ovulation and fertility (and, therefore, progesterone production). They are primarily intended to raise progesterone levels in relation to estrogen. Plants like Dioscorea villosa and Tribulus Terrestris are examples of those that contain saponins. Enhancing the ovarian tissue's sensitivity or responsiveness to the activity of the gonadotrophins may serve as an alternate method of action.

Hormones and menstrual cycles are positively regulated by linseed meals in a number of ways. The precursors in linseed meals are converted in the intestinal system into the lignans enterodiol and enterolactone. In women with regular menstrual cycles, linseed meal has been shown to improve ovulation rates and lengthen the luteal phase. Despite not raising luteal phase progesterone levels, flaxseed (linseed) meal does raise luteal phase progesterone levels relative to estradiol.

It's also important to address the secondary causes of anovulation and/or relative progesterone deficiency, such as stress, which can be treated with nervine tonics, sedatives, and adaptogens; low body weight, which can be treated with the right diet; excessive exercise, which should be reduced; and other metabolic or hormonal conditions, such as thyroid disorders, which can be treated with medical, herbal, or dietary intervention.

In addition to using magnesium, vitamin B6, vitamin E, evening primrose oil, and vitamin B6 to treat progesterone deficient symptoms.

Some medical professionals advise using progesterone that is "natural" or "bio-identical." These are a form of hormone replacement, and they don't address the underlying issues that lead to progesterone deficiency disorders. In reality, the body's attempts to release progesterone are likely to be reduced as a result of the feedback reaction, which occurs when endogenous hormone levels fall in the presence of replacement hormones. The choice to replace any hormone, whether natural or synthetic, must be based on the intended results. Herbal remedies may be more effective for women trying to resolve issues by restoring normal hormone levels; those interested in symptom control may want to try progesterone or herbs, and those who have tried herbal remedies but were unable to restore a regular cycle may want to think about hormonal remedies to protect the endometrium. In any situation, it is advised to seek the counsel of a specialist in this field.

ANDROGENS

Androgens, a group of male and female hormones, have a masculinizing impact. Although androgen levels in women are typically much lower than in males, certain medical diseases can cause elevated androgen levels in women, which can cause irregular menstruation or amenorrhea. Alternately, decreased androgen levels may contribute to several of the symptoms typically linked to the menopausal transition.

ANDROGEN EXCESS

Causes

Excess androgen production can result from a variety of gynecological and other disorders.

- Ovarian causes: Hyperthecosis, androgen-producing ovarian tumors, and polycystic ovarian syndrome.
- Adrenal gland disorders: Adrenal gland tumors that produce androgen include congenital or adult-onset adrenal hyperplasia.
- Drugs: Some medications have hydrogenizing effects and can affect the menstrual flow and cycle regularity: The progestogens phenytoin sodium (Dilantin), dydrogesterone (Duphaston), and danazol (Danocrine), as well as the corticosteroids and corticotrophins, and anabolic steroids like Deca-Durabolin.
- Metabolic and hormonal states: Obesity, post-menopause, and Cushing's syndrome.

Signs and symptoms

Excessive hair growth, also known as hirsutism, or excessive scalp hair loss, also known as androgenic alopecia, are the most prevalent effects of increased androgens. Elevated androgen levels can exacerbate acne or even create it, and in premenopausal women, amenorrhea or irregular menstruation can also happen.

When coarse hair develops on the chin, upper lip, cheeks, around the nipples, and in between the breasts, the buttocks, the lower back, and the lower belly, it is known as hirsutism, also known as male-pattern hair growth. However, not all cases of hirsutism are brought on by elevated testosterone levels, and both the quantity and distribution of hair are genetic traits. Women with darker hair and eyes typically have more body hair than women with lighter skin tones or Asian women.

Acne and/or increased male-pattern hair growth during puberty, along with delayed menarche, are indications of androgen excess. In women who have passed menarche, changes in the amount and coarseness of body or facial hair, particularly when this is also accompanied by menstrual irregularity, are indications of androgen excess.

Another symptom of androgen excess that can appear in pre-or post-menopausal women is androgenic alopecia. Additionally called male-pattern baldness. The scalp may experience a broad thinning of hair or only experience it at the crown. The pace of hair loss varies, and typically, the hair gets finer and thinner. There isn't baldness all over. Even when their testosterone levels are not noticeably increased above normal, menopausal women can experience androgenic alopecia, facial acne, and hair growth. This is hypothesized to be caused by a decrease in estrogen levels, which diminish SHBG, as well as an increase in adrenal androgens or an enhanced sensitivity to them.

Rare cases of extreme androgen excess or virilization manifest as clitoris enlargement and diminished breast size. Extremely high androgen levels are typically caused by androgen-producing cancers of the ovary or adrenal gland. Some medications, like danazol, can potentially virilize people.

Diagnosis

The first step is to perform tests to check for high levels of SHBG, the carrier protein, and serum testosterone. The strongest predictor of ovarian androgen synthesis is serum testosterone, while SHBG indicates the amount of free testosterone that is available for androgenizing effects. Another indicator of androgen activity is the free androgen index (FAI), which measures unbound androgens. In polycystic ovarian syndrome and androgen-producing ovarian tumors, ovarian androgen production is increased.

When adult-onset adrenal hyperplasia or androgen-producing adrenal tumors are suspected, DHEA sulfate is the most accurate test for determining aberrant adrenal androgen levels. Women with adult-onset adrenal hyperplasia frequently experience hirsutism, low height, high blood pressure, and irregular menstrual cycles.

Androgen levels are frequently within the normal range in those with hirsutism, acne, or male-pattern baldness, and the issue appears to result from an inherent sensitivity to androgens in the pilosebaceous unit. The same approach should be taken whether the androgen levels are elevated or more sensitive than usual.

THE MEDICAL APPROACH

The reasons for androgen excess must be addressed before treating it. Weight loss is necessary for obesity, and modest doses of dexamethasone are used to treat congenital adrenal hyperplasia and adult-onset adrenal hyperplasia. HRT is frequently administered to postmenopausal women (a type of corticosteroid). Usually, malignancies of the ovary or the adrenal gland must be removed. It is possible to prescribe estrogen to raise SHBG levels.

Aldactone (spironolactone), Androcur (cyproterone acetate), or the Pill known as Diane, which contains a small quantity of cyproterone acetate, are the three most frequently prescribed drugs for hirsutism. By inhibiting the androgens' ability to interact with tissues that are typically receptive to androgens (such as the skin and hair follicles), pharmaceuticals like Aldactone, Androcur, and Diane reduce the effects of androgens. These medications do this by blocking receptor sites on the cells. Some of the new "third-generation" Pills (Femoden, Marvelon, Minulet, Triminulet, and Trioden) contain the progestogens norgestimate, desogestrel, and gestodene and have a low androgen potency. These sorts of Pills, however, may not be appropriate for all women as their use can increase the risk of blood clot formation.

When hirsutism medication regimens are stopped, the hair frequently grows back, and the medication may need to be taken for a long time in order to effectively control the condition. Many oral contraceptives contain the progestogen levonorgestrel, which has androgenizing effects and is frequently inappropriate for women with excess androgen. When contraception is required, and testosterone excess is a problem, a gynecologist should be consulted to decide which Pill is appropriate. The Pill's androgenic potential is also influenced by the number of progestogens being consumed. Triphasil and Tranquiller, for instance, which have low doses of levonorgestrel, typically do not increase symptoms of androgen excess.

THE NATURAL THERAPIST'S APPROACH

Once more, the treatment is determined by the reason. Advice is necessary for women with the polycystic ovarian syndrome (PCOS) in order to treat insulin resistance, maintain hormonal balance, and resume normal menstruation. In order to counteract the masculinizing effects of androgens, post-menopausal women can employ vegetarian diets and phytoestrogens to raise SHBG (which declines along with the fall in estrogen levels). If at all possible, androgenizing drug users should be recommended to their general practitioner to consider changing their medication.

It can be challenging to manage excessive male pattern hair growth or hair loss linked to excess androgen. It has been demonstrated that Serenoa repens can treat hirsutism and also helps with androgenic alopecia. By inhibiting androgens from connecting with cell receptor sites, Turnera aphrodisiacal and the Smilax species (sarsaparilla) may be able to counteract the effects of androgens. Competitive inhibition is the term for this. They are not as dependable or as quick to work as medications. The most effective combination can be pharmaceuticals initially, followed by herbal therapies to preserve the status quo when excessive hair growth or loss is a major issue.

Another strategy is to accelerate the aromatization of androgens into estrogens. The aromatization process is accelerated by Glycyrrhiza glabra, and specifically by paeoniflorin, a Paeonia lactiflora component, which lowers testosterone levels. Traditional Chinese medicine's Peony and Liquorice Combination is effective for excessive ovarian androgen production; however, its effects are frequently transient.

When women are obese or have PCOS, losing weight or maintaining a healthy weight will help to regulate androgen levels. This can be accomplished with regular meals, a low-fat diet, and carbs with a low glycemic index. Exercise in the morning, such as brisk walking or repeated sets of weightlifting exercises that raise the heart rate, also speeds up weight loss. Diets rich in fiber and phytoestrogens, which bind to androgens and render them mostly inaccessible, help people lose weight and boost their levels of SHBG.

When androgenic alopecia or excessive hair growth are the main issues, treatment must be continued for several months and, in some cases, forever. It is crucial that the chosen treatments are deemed secure for long-term use. Self-treatment is not appropriate for this illness. Advice from a professional with expertise in this field is crucial.

ANDROGEN DEFICIENCY

Recently, the term female androgen deficiency syndrome has been coined to characterize a series of symptoms seen in women that are thought to be linked to low testosterone levels. Low libido with diminished sexual desire, ongoing, unexplained exhaustion, and a lower sense of well-being in conjunction with pubic hair thinning or loss are the hallmarks of this illness. Muscle mass loss and a decline in assertiveness might come next. Even when a woman is receiving sufficient estrogen replacement therapy, androgen deficiency syndrome symptoms might still manifest.

The symptoms typically appear gradually and can appear as early as the late thirties because the drop in androgens typically begins much earlier than menopause. Because the ovaries suddenly stop producing testosterone, symptoms are more severe in women who have had their ovaries surgically removed.

Women who experience early ovarian failure may also experience symptoms of androgen insufficiency syndrome. Testosterone shortage may result from ovarian failure brought on by the administration of GnRH agonists for the treatment of endometriosis or fibroids, as well as after chemotherapy or radiotherapy. Due to the suppression of ACTH caused by corticosteroid use, adrenal androgen production can be decreased.

Relative androgen deficiency can also result from estrogen therapy. It has been demonstrated that oral estrogens, such as those found in the oral contraceptive pill (OCP) or used in hormone replacement treatment reduce the levels of free testosterone in the blood. The Pill boosts SHBG while decreasing ovarian androgen production. When using the Pill, women in their late reproductive years may have symptoms of reduced libido that are linked to both the Pill and age-related falling testosterone levels.

After starting HRT, postmenopausal women may experience the symptoms of androgen shortage. This is linked to a reduction in the stimulus for post-menopausal ovarian thecal testosterone production due to a replacement estrogen-induced increase in SHBG and pituitary LH secretion.

Diagnosis

Clinical evaluation and biochemical tests serve as the foundation for diagnosis. The biochemical parameters of total testosterone, SHBG, and free androgen index are advised (FAI). Current testosterone tests are made to assess testosterone levels in men within their normal range. The typical testosterone level in post-menopausal women has not yet been determined, and there are no recognized criteria, such as the free testosterone level, with a set threshold below which this syndrome can be identified by the results of blood tests. Additionally, the common tests used to measure testosterone levels in reproductive females at the lower end of the normal range are notoriously unreliable and do not distinguish between low and mid-normal levels. The androgen status is thought to be more effectively reflected by a "sensitive" testosterone level. In order to prevent a falsely low reading, blood should be drawn for testing before noon and after day seven in menstrual women.

Women with the typical symptoms of androgen insufficiency syndrome who have total testosterone levels below 2 nmol/L and normal or higher SHBG levels may be diagnosed with the condition until extremely sensitive assays are routinely available.

THE MEDICAL APPROACH

A tablet, injection, implant, transdermal patch, or gel can be used to provide testosterone. In clinical studies involving women, the majority of these medicines' efficacy and safety have not been shown. In Western Australia, there is a cream with 1 percent testosterone available for women; however, there is no long-term research on its use or how the absorption may change depending on where the cream is applied. In modest, short-term research, pre-menopausal women with low libido and low testosterone had an improvement in their general well-being, mood, and sexual function.

It is preferable to restore testosterone levels to the upper end of the normal physiological range for young ovulating women in order to achieve a successful treatment response in terms of improved desire. Before starting testosterone therapy, symptomatic post-menopausal women on oral estrogen therapy who have a normal testosterone level but a high SHBG and a low free androgen index should switch to non-oral medication. After six to eight weeks, another blood test and a clinical evaluation are required to determine whether testosterone therapy is still required. The requirement for testosterone therapy may also be eliminated if these women stop taking their estrogen supplements.

Women may be concerned about the masculinizing side effects of androgen replacement therapy, such as acne, hirsutism, voice deepening, and increased libido, which might result in unwanted symptoms.

THE NATURAL THERAPIST'S APPROACH

Because of the relative newness of the diagnosis of "female androgen insufficiency syndrome," there are no clear therapy recommendations. A woman with symptoms resembling this condition is typically recommended to adopt stress-reduction strategies, engage in regular exercise, and consume a healthy diet. As suggested by additional symptoms, herbal tonics, adaptogens, and/or nervine tonics are administered.

7

Natural Ways To Balance
Your Hormones

If everyone had access to a mystical Shangri-La where gorgeous fruits and vegetables appeared out of thin air in their immaculate gardens, where there were no worries about money or family issues, where they had unlimited time and energy to participate in Zumba classes and bike around picturesque lakes under clear skies, and where their skin and lips were shielded from all artificial chemicals while maintaining a healthy weight, But alas, in the actual world, your fertility cycle is a complex feedback system that is influenced by a variety of outside influences that might upset your equilibrium. Because of this, your cycles frequently reflect both your general health and fertility. Therefore, your hormones may be out of balance if you suffer any of the following: poor diet, stress, lack of exercise, lack of sleep, being underweight or overweight, perimenopause, mood swings, insomnia, or symptoms of menopause (hot flashes, night sweats, and vaginal dryness).

You can naturally balance your hormones in essentially two ways. The first is done entirely on your own, while the second is done under the direction of any number of natural health care practitioners. In any case, the greatest way to see the procedure is as active nurturing as opposed to denying your body. Although it may appear like semantic games, the brain is a strong tool. Instead of focusing on how much you are starving yourself by forgoing chocolate cake, try to consider how much you are nourishing your body by eating things like fresh fruits and vegetables. Who am I kidding? Oh hell? Although it might be challenging, the benefits, particularly for those who are trying to get pregnant, will more than makeup for any feeling of deprivation.

MAKING HEALTHY CHANGES ON YOUR OWN

The recommendations listed below give you an overview of the kinds of things you can frequently perform without ever visiting a clinic.

Herbal supplements

Perhaps no herb is as well regarded as Vitex among those that are currently frequently used to treat women's hormonal problems. It is a complex herb that is frequently regarded as the most significant all-natural treatment for ailments brought on by hormone imbalance, including PMS, perimenopause, and everything in between. It is thought to be particularly potent because it especially affects the hormonal loop connecting the hypothalamus, pituitary, and ovaries, the trifecta of women's bodies. In reality, the majority of practitioners of natural medicine now quite routinely advise Vitex.

Unfortunately, there hasn't been as much research done on Vitex or herbs in general as there has been for conventional pharmaceuticals, despite the fact that several scientific studies support its effectiveness and safety in treating a variety of hormonal disorders. This is due in part to the high cost of completing clinical studies as well as the fact that producers of herbal supplements have little motivation to spend money on research because their goods are rarely patentable. Additionally, you should be aware that the FDA does not control herbs, so people should utilize these treatments with caution.

I advise you to utilize them at first under the supervision of an expert in the field. This is partially due to the sheer number of herb variations (which are frequently aggressively advertised!), but herbs can only be safe and successful if the right herb and dosage are carefully chosen for the particular illness you're attempting to treat. Regardless, there is a ton of in-depth information available thanks to the numerous websites that are specifically focused on this subject. I would only trust websites that are run by credible medical professionals, nurses, dietitians, or other experts in women's health.

Diet

The famous Harvard Nurses' Health Study from the 1990s, which tracked 18,000 women's diets for eight years to identify which foods enhanced their fertility, is one of the most significant research in this area. The suggestions below may also be applicable to you if your cycles are in any way irregular and you are not currently attempting to conceive. Women who have PCOS are the only exception. The Fertility Diet, a 2009 book by Harvard researchers, contains a detailed discussion of all the recommendations they made based on their findings. A summary of some of their findings is provided below:

- Avoid trans fats. Read your labels! "Hydrogenated oils" is another term for trans fats. This type of fat can harm your heart and blood vessels as well as impair your fertility.
- Add additional polyunsaturated fats to your diet. Two factors that are beneficial for fertility are increased

insulin sensitivity and decreased inflammation, both of which can be improved by consuming monounsaturated and polyunsaturated fats. Enjoy nuts, seeds, and cold-water fish such as salmon and sardines. And, of course, decrease saturated fats.

- Increase vegetable protein. Try to replace a serving of meat each day with a variety of vegetable proteins such as beans, peas, soybeans, tofu, and nuts.
- Choose slowly digested carbs. You can enhance your fertility by eating a diet rich in fiber-rich foods, including fresh fruits and vegetables, whole grains, and beans.
- Get plenty of iron from plants. This includes whole-grain cereals as well as spinach, tomatoes, beets, beans, and pumpkin.
- Drink a lot of water to stay hydrated. You don't need to avoid everything else, and even coffee and tea are fine in moderation. But skip sugary sodas when you are trying to conceive.
- Take a multivitamin. If you are trying to get pregnant, be sure to take at least 400 micrograms a day of folic acid to help prevent spinal cord defects in the baby.

Achieving an Ideal Body Fat Ratio

The optimum BMI range for healthy ovulation is between 20 and 24 points. Extra estrogen production brought on by being overweight can seriously disrupt your intricate hormonal feedback system. However, being underweight can completely stop your ovulation.

Exercise

Use any activity that motivates you to work out, whether it's biking, swimming, or something else that doesn't feel like a job. Finding something to look forward to rather than detest is the key. So, 15 laps of jogging around an indoor track each day? Not really.

Stress Reduction

One of the nicest things you can do when trying to regulate your hormones is the innovative idea of pampering yourself, sticking with the theme of nurturing rather than depriving. That entails, among other things, choosing activities you enjoy above simply engaging in what is considered calming by society if you want to reduce stress. Therefore, if practicing yoga or meditation sounds like your notion of a painfully slow death from boredom, consider hiking, reading a great book, or taking a hot bath instead.

Sleep

Sleep for at least eight hours! Even better if it means TIVOing Jimmy Fallon so you can watch him on your stationary cycle the next morning.

Night Lighting

What makes women who wake up to use the bathroom and then stumble into furniture in the dark different from those who, because of all the extra light in their bedrooms, can almost see the tiny warning labels on prescription bottles? Obviously, the caliber of their cycles! It turns out that the pineal gland detects tiny amounts of light that slip through our eyelids as we sleep from seemingly harmless sources like the moon, a nightlight, or even a digital clock.

The issue is that this gland secretes melatonin, which has an impact on the hypothalamus, the nucleus of a woman's world. Therefore, you might want to try totally blocking off any source of light if you are experiencing issues with your cycles, which can range from irregularity to brief luteal phases. (To do this, blackout curtains may need to be used to block off light from the outside.)

Avoiding Hormone Disruptors

It's unlikely that you will be able to totally avoid hormone disruptors known as xenohormones, which are synthetic compounds with the capacity to, well, disrupt your hormones unless you live in a cave! A class of preservatives called parabens, which is included in common goods like makeup and shampoos as well as foods and beverages, is among the most pervasive and possibly dangerous. Phthalates, another class of chemical compounds typically found in flexible plastic, are linked to endocrine disruption. To prevent harmful chemicals from entering your kitchen and medicine cabinet, attempt to find replacement goods that do not contain them. Obviously, you can't avoid them entirely, but you might want to attempt to concentrate on the ones that you can easily keep out of your own house.

Dealing with Thyroid Disorders

One of the glands that control most bodily activities is the thyroid. An underactive thyroid can have a disastrous effect on a woman's periods and her health. Fortunately, women who chart have the edge over non-charters in that they frequently have the ability to identify potential issues by simply examining the pattern of their waking temperatures.

The first sign that they may have hypothyroidism is frequently abnormally low temperatures (in the low 96s and low 97s pre-ovulatory), although temperatures by themselves are insufficient. Ask to have a thyroid blood test that evaluates free T3, free T4, and TPO in addition to TSH and T4 if you experience low temperatures along with any of the additional symptoms listed below. Because the latter three are frequently not evaluated as part of a standard blood work panel, you might need to be more assertive in the case of the latter three.

The following are some of the most typical signs of a thyroid disorder:

- Infertility
- PMS
- Low libido
- Heavy, prolonged, or painful menses
- Short luteal phases or other signs of luteal phase issues
- Prolonged, less-fertile-quality cervical fluid
- Long or irregular cycles

- Anovulation

Many of the dietary and lifestyle recommendations in this chapter can aid in improved thyroid function.

Luteal Phase Problems

As you've read, progesterone is released during the luteal phase after ovulation. Ideally, you want it to be between 12 and 16 days, whether you are trying to conceive or not (or just living your life!). This will allow you more time to enjoy your infertility if you want to avoid becoming pregnant, and it's important for the fertilized egg to have enough time to implant in the uterus if you want to get pregnant.

There are a few natural remedies you might consider if charting reveals that you do, in fact, have a luteal phase that is too short. Major expert on the topic Marilyn Shannon, author of Fertility, Cycles, and Nutrition, thinks that luteal phase deficiencies are closely associated with PMS. She advises Optivite PMT or ProCycle PMS as a supplement, as well as increasing flax and/or fish oil intake. Additionally, think about the herbal supplements mentioned earlier in this chapter.

Working With a Complementary Health Practitioner

Previously, any healthcare professionals who had not received their education from conventional medical colleges were referred to as "alternative" and were believed to be engaged in voodoo science. However, because so many individuals report such wonderful outcomes, there is a more favorable acceptance of certified complementary health practitioners today. They either practice independently, collaboratively with other natural health professionals in a clinic or with traditional physicians utilizing complementary or integrative methods.

Nevertheless, not all medical disorders may be treated as effectively by Western traditional medicine alone. Nutritionists, who are currently regarded as mainstream, as well as complementary practitioners like naturopaths, acupuncturists, Chinese herbal medicine experts, and even conventional doctors who also use more natural modalities, maybe the best specialists to consult with in the case of balancing women's hormones. The fundamental tenet that unites all of these strategies is that it is frequently preferable to adopt non-invasive, efficient, but gentle methods of treating women's health issues rather than relying on potent medications and invasive procedures that frequently result in unwanted side effects. The majority of these professionals will use a range of therapies, including acupuncture, bio-identical hormones, herbal supplements, and other physical therapies. What is best for each woman will depend on her particular set of circumstances (for example, a woman with PCOS will be best treated by following certain protocols in diet and lifestyle that may be very different from a woman who is dealing with PMS). However, depending on your circumstances, I would advise you to further investigate this subject on your own, as being hormonally unbalanced can negatively affect your fertility as well as your general health.

Bio-identical hormones

The usage of truly natural, or bio-identical, hormones rather than the synthetic varieties created by pharmaceutical firms in a lab, according to many experts, is the key to hormone balance. These bio-identicals are derived from plants, like soy and wild yams, but their molecular makeup is exactly the same as that of the progesterone and estrogens produced by female bodies.

They come in a variety of forms, including pills, patches, and different vaginal creams. Additionally, there are specialized estrogen and progesterone blends made by different compounding pharmacies. In addition, younger women can also benefit from hormones if they have irregular cycles, few or no periods, or other indicators of a hormonal imbalance. This is true even though both bio-identical and synthetic hormone therapies are linked to the treatment of menopausal symptoms like vaginal dryness and hot flashes.

You should be aware; however, that hormonal therapy of any kind is a very complex subject. While it is true that many doctors and other health professionals assert that bio-identical hormones are safer, more effective, and have fewer side effects than synthetic hormones, all of these claims are vigorously contested by other members of the medical profession. In any case, if this is a choice that appeals to you, you should be aware that even proponents of bio-identical hormones will tell you that if you want to use them to balance your own hormones, you must collaborate closely with a physician or other healthcare provider in order to carefully assess your needs and customize your treatment.

THE BEST WAY TO GET IN BALANCE

If you're one of the fortunate people for whom this chapter has no application, fantastic! For everyone else, you should only be aware that there are many easy, affordable, and noninvasive ways to naturally balance your hormones before turning to any intensive medical procedures. This shouldn't come as a surprise because a nutrient-rich whole food diet, regular exercise, keeping a healthy weight, and stress management techniques are the foundation of all healthy life. The main takeaway from this chapter is that a woman's total health, not only her ability to conceive, is reflected in her hormonal balance. As a result, you should make an effort to encourage and uphold a healthy lifestyle by taking the necessary personal steps.

8

Prostaglandins: Maintaining The Orderly Function Of The Reproductive Organs

The broad family of hormone-like compounds known as eicosanoids, which also include prostaglandins, leukotriene, and thromboxane, regulates ovulation, menstruation, labor, as well as many other non-gynecological events. When one group of eicosanoids triggers muscle spasm, another group balances that action by triggering relaxation; similarly, when blood clotting is induced, a balancing anti-clotting response is also produced.

However, occasionally, production will prefer one or more family members over the others due to a number of variables such as illness, inflammation, allergy, hormone fluctuations, or a bad diet. These imbalances are thought to play a role in common gynecological symptoms such as period discomfort, heavy periods, PMS, and endometriosis. They may be transitory or persistent.

The prostaglandins family is similar to an extended clan made up of smaller nuclear-style family-like units. The prostacyclin and thromboxane families, as well as a collection of distinct prostaglandins, are among these families. All of the members of a big family have a wide range of duties to do. Prostaglandins, for instance, affect blood clotting, muscle activity, and inflammatory reactions all across the body, whereas thromboxanes affect blood clotting and blood vessel activity.

Each extended eicosanoid clan has a letter of the alphabet used to identify its members. So, for instance, TX A, a member of the thromboxane family and a member of the A branch, is responsible for the clumping together of platelets. The acronym LT B refers to the leukotriene from its family's B branch, which is in charge of luring white blood cells to inflamed regions.

PG E is one of the prostaglandins; however, there are other others as well. Each member of the thromboxane, prostaglandin and leukotriene families has a specific job. Like every family, some family members tend to be annoyed while others are more helpful. As an illustration, one leukotriene may initiate certain inflammatory processes while another, either a distant or close clan member, will act as a soothing agent.

The names of the various prostaglandins, thromboxane, and leukotriene are then given series numbers to aid in identifying what each clan member does, what they are made of, and how they appear.

- Series 1 is anti-inflammatory, relaxes muscles and is derived from two fatty acids known as linoleic acid and gamma-linoleic acid.
- Series 2 and 4 come from arachidonic acid, found in the cell membranes of animals, and are largely pro-inflammatory.
- Series 3 and 5 reduce abnormal blood clotting and are anti-inflammatory, and are made from eicosapentaenoic acid (EPA).

THE KEY PLAYERS IN THE MENSTRUAL CYCLE

Prostaglandins E, series 2 (PGE 2)

Most bodily tissues make PGE 2, which is abundant in the ovarian follicle, the uterus, and the brain. PGE 2 prevents platelets from adhering to one another and widens blood vessels in the endometrium, increasing menstrual blood loss. PGE 2 promotes relaxation in the Fallopian tube while dramatically increasing muscular contraction in the uterine muscle.

Prostaglandins F, series 2 (PGF 2α)

PGF 2 (the alpha describes this prostaglandin's structure to a biochemist) rises as the menstrual cycle proceeds, probably because estrogen and progesterone have an impact on its synthesis. PGF 2 causes blood vessels in the endometrium to contract, which is the reverse of what PGE 2 does. Both PGF 2 and PGE 2 elicit muscle spasms in the myometrium, and both are increased in women who have dysmenorrhea.

Prostaglandins E, series 1 (PGE 1)

The so-called "good" prostaglandin is PGE 1. It also promotes salt excretion, relaxes blood vessels, reduces inflammation, enhances the action of insulin, and controls calcium metabolism, among other crucial roles. It also prevents platelets from clumping. PGE 1's precise function in the reproductive system is still unknown. In the luteal phase, it is thought to have a hormone-regulating effect that is most pronounced. It might also lessen the prolactin sensitivity of the tissue.

Prostacyclin, series 2 (PGI 2)

The uterus, ovarian follicles, corpus luteum, and the walls of arteries all produce the hormone prostacyclin (PGI 2). It relaxes the uterine muscle, widens blood channels, and prevents platelets from clumping together. The opposing action on blood arteries and platelets is caused by thromboxane 2 (TXA 2). It causes blood vessel constriction and platelet clumping. PGF 2 has the opposite impact on uterine muscle than PGI 2, causing it to contract.

Leukotriene

Leukotriene generally increases uterine contraction, and dysmenorrhea women have higher levels of leukotriene families C and D. White blood cells are drawn to inflamed tissues by leukotriene B (LTB 4), which is higher in endometriosis-affected women and may also play a role in breast cancer.

THE OMEGA-6 AND OMEGA-3 PATHWAYS

The many prostaglandins, thromboxane, and leukotriene are produced in response to complicated stimuli. The ratio of each of the several series created depends on more than just the building blocks of essential fatty acids. A number of other biochemical and organ-specific processes, such as menstruation, also influence the sequence of prostaglandins, etc., to be created. Tissues manufacture eicosanoids in reaction to a stimulus—inflammation, for example.

The omega-6 and omega-3 routes are the two processes by which dietary fatty acids are transformed into fatty acids that act as eicosanoids' substrates.

The omega-6 pathway

The important fatty acid linoleic acid, which is a significant component of many seed and vegetable oils, as well as the majority of nuts, organ meats, and human milk, is the first step in the omega-6 pathway. The amounts of linoleic acid in dairy products and coconut oil are extremely low.

Gamma- and linoleic acids are abundant in evening primrose oil, blackcurrant seed oil, and starflower seed oil (GLA). By specifically raising levels of dihomogamma-linolenic acid, these beneficial supplements can expedite the development of the series 1 prostaglandin (DGLA). These seed oils contain a variety of advantageous qualities. In addition to having anti-inflammatory properties that can lessen the severity of eczema, asthma, and allergies, they also prevent blood clotting, lower cholesterol, and have vasodilatory effects. They also have a significant modulatory role in the immune system.

Arachidonic acid, which is produced from linoleic acid or taken in as part of the food, is a precursor for the synthesis of series 2 prostaglandins, thromboxane, and series 4 leukotriene and is also a component of the omega-6 pathway. This fatty acid can be found in human breast milk as well as other animal products like meat and eggs. Since it may be produced from linoleic acid, arachidonic acid is not a necessary fatty acid.

It is thought that altering the starting ingredients' concentrations (linoleic acid, GLA, and arachidonic acid) can alter the ratio of series 1 to series 2 prostaglandins. Both the inflammatory and anti-inflammatory series (series 1 and series 2) may be created if food sources are largely from the linoleic acid end of the route. However, pro-inflammatory series 2 effects will be preferred if arachidonic-containing foods are the focus of the diet.

The omega-3 pathway

Alpha-linoleic acid, an important fatty acid, is the initial step in the production of omega-3 fatty acids. Dark green leafy vegetables, walnut and canola seed oils, soybean oil, linseed and canola seed oils contain it. Alpha-linoleic acid undergoes the same series of enzymatic processes as the omega-6 pathway to become eicosapentaenoic acid (EPA) and docosahexaenoic acid (DHA). The production of series 3 prostaglandins, thromboxane, and series 5 leukotriene is selectively increased by the creation of EPA. Because arachidonic acid and EPA compete for the same enzyme to produce their respective end products, EPA functions as a competitive inhibitor in the conversion of arachidonic acid to the series 2 and 4 eicosanoids. For instance, when both arachidonic acid and EPA are present, a balance of pro and anti-inflammatory, anti-thrombotic and blood-clotting, muscle relaxing and muscle contracting eicosanoids are generated.

DHA, the final component of the omega-3 pathway, inhibits the creation of series 2 and 4 eicosanoids and, unlike EPA, does not act as a substrate for eicosanoid synthesis.

A lengthy number of therapeutic benefits of EPA and DHA can be found, including a decrease in platelet stickiness and the risk of cardiovascular disease, a reduction in inflammation in disorders like arthritis, and an improvement in allergic reaction-related conditions like asthma and eczema. Additionally, these oils have the potential to treat gynecological issues.

It does not appear that humans easily convert the alpha-linolenic acid present in seeds and seed oils into EPA, which acts as a substrate for the advantageous series 3 prostaglandins. The levels of EPA increased greater in the fish oil group when volunteers followed a low-fat diet and supplemented with either linseed oil or fish oils. The amount of linoleic acid in the diet affects the conversion of alpha-linolenic acid from seeds, and lower intakes of omega-6 fatty acids, particularly linoleic acid, resulting in higher conversion rates. For those aiming to prevent or treat cardiovascular disease, oily, cold-water fish oils appear to be the most helpful. They may also show to be more therapeutically advantageous for gynecological symptoms that respond to increased levels of EPA.

An alternate supply of EPA for the synthesis of prostaglandins, thromboxane, and leukotriene is found in fish oils. The cold-water and oilier fish and shellfish are the best nutritional sources. As dietary supplements, fish oils are also offered in tablet form.

Fatty acids for gynecological complaints

GLA

The GLA found in evening primrose and other seed oils, as well as fish oils, appear to have a positive effect on a number of gynecological issues. However, meals that elevate series 2 prostaglandins selectively should be avoided wherever feasible to provide the optimum therapeutic benefits.

Menorrhagia

Arachidonic acid levels are greater than normal, and the production of prostaglandins E2 is enhanced in women with menorrhagia (PGE 2). As a result, blood coagulation is compromised, blood vessels are dilated, and abnormal bleeding occurs. Prostaglandins F2 (PGF 2) are normally transformed from PGE 2 into prostaglandins F2 (PGF 2); however, this conversion is decreased in women with menorrhagia. Prostacyclin 2 levels are also elevated in these women (PGI 2). As a blood artery dilatation agent and blood coagulation inhibitor, PGI 2 has been shown to increase menstrual bleeding. Medications that inhibit the production of prostaglandins into PGI 2 include Naprogesic and Ponstan.

Menstrual bleeding may be lessened by reducing dietary fat intake, increasing consumption of omega-3-rich foods, and taking fish oil or GLA supplements. Both of these oils have the ability to lower PGE 2 levels in certain tissues. Estrogen and maybe arachidonic acid synthesis may be reduced by reducing dietary fat intake. PGE 2 and PGI 2 synthesis may also be stimulated by a relative excess of estrogen. Women who follow a low-fat diet report that their periods are lighter, but a study has not been done to determine the primary causes responsible for this shift.

Dysmenorrhea

Menstruating women have higher levels of prostaglandins 2 and 2, which may help explain the symptoms of primary dysmenorrhea, such as increased uterine muscle contraction, reduced blood flow to the uterus, and lowered pain threshold. These changes in prostaglandins production may help explain these symptoms.

Because it occurs more frequently and is alleviated by the Pill during ovulatory cycles, dysmenorrhea may be linked to the manufacture of the eicosanoids that cause muscle spasms. Progesterone levels affect prostaglandins' ability to cause uterine spasms in the uterus, and high levels make the uterus resistant to this effect. Menstruation-related symptoms such as dysmenorrhea are brought on by a drop in progesterone levels.

Primary dysmenorrhea may also be caused by leukotriene. Those leukotrienes (C4 and D4) that increase uterine muscle spasm in women with severe dysmenorrhea are elevated in these women's blood; a diet rich in oily fish and avoiding foods high in arachidonic acid (meat, liver, and kidney) reduces the severity of dysmenorrhea and improves the synthesis of series 3 prostaglandin and leukotriene.

When traditional prostaglandin-inhibiting medicines have failed to relieve dysmenorrhea, fish oils appear to be very helpful (which do not inhibit the production of leukotriene). Dysmenorrhea is reduced in women using fish oils at doses of between 2000 and 3000 mg per day.

The pain of dysmenorrhea can be alleviated by using evening primrose oil. Series 1 prostaglandin levels improved, and series 2 prostaglandins decreased, but the reasons for this are not known. Despite these alterations, no research has examined them in relation to dysmenorrhea. Doses ranging from 1000 mg daily for ten days prior to menstruation to 3000 mg daily for the entire month have been shown to reduce discomfort.

Hormonal imbalance

It's been hypothesized that PMS is brought on by an imbalance in the body's production of prostaglandins, which are chemicals generated in the brain, breast, digestive tract, kidney, and reproductive tract. Oestrogen and progesterone (relative excess of estrogen) could be contributing components to this imbalance. Side effects and cautions accompany drugs that successfully modify or inhibit prostaglandins, which have been demonstrated to alleviate PMS.

In addition to alleviating PMS symptoms, GLA-rich food supplements such as evening primrose oil and starflower oil are safe and effective alternatives to synthetic hormone replacement therapy. In theory, this would lessen the overactive effects of prolactin by increasing levels of PGE 1; however clinical trials have failed to demonstrate any benefit in alleviating the symptoms of PMS.

Taking between 3000 and 4000 mg of evening primrose oil daily for the duration of the cycle has been shown to be helpful in the treatment of PMS, but it must be used in conjunction with a diet low in animal (saturated) fats and a higher intake of omega-3 fatty acids for the greatest outcomes. Getting the desired outcomes from supplements often needs a longer period of time than the standard three months.

Endometriosis

Prostaglandin and leukotriene imbalances in women with endometriosis have a negative impact on ovulation and fertility as well as on embryo development and tube motility. Dysmenorrhoea severity may also be influenced by prostaglandins and leukotrienes, two more inflammatory hormones.

PGF 2 levels are higher in endometriosis patients, although PGE 2 levels are lower. Increased levels of PGF 2 may be a factor in the sensation of pain. LTB 4 (also known as leukotriene B) draws white blood cells to inflamed sites and is increased in women with endometriosis. Sperm, ovum, or the embryo's development may be hampered by the white cells' increased activity, which has been linked to infertility.

To test the effects of DHA and EPA in the treatment of endometriosis in rabbits, researchers fed the animals fish oils. Fish oils appear to be useful in treating both inflammation and severity of endometriosis, as PGE 2 and PGF 2 levels did not increase, and the amount of endometriosis decreased.

For infertility, GLA and fish oils may inhibit the development of LTB 4. Fish and evening primrose oil may also improve the ratio of PGE 1 to PGE 2 in white blood cells, which may reduce inflammation and increase fertility.

Fish oils, rather than evening primrose oils, may be more beneficial for women with endometriosis who are experiencing dysmenorrhea or reproductive issues (or similar). Recommendations range between 2000 and 4000 mg of this drug daily.

Benign and malignant breast changes

The leukotriene LTB 4 may have a role in the development of breast cancers, and supplements including linseed oil or fish oils have been proven to suppress tumor growth and metastasis in animal tests. As far as I know, this has no practical use for women.

Premenstrual discomfort, swelling, and increased nodularity are thought to be linked to the inflammatory changes brought on by prostaglandins, which are responsible for benign breast alterations. Increased heat and inflammation in the breast have been proven to be caused by PGE 2, and vasodilation has been observed.

The synthesis of inflammatory prostaglandins may rise when estrogen and progesterone are out of balance, according to prior research. Prolactin-induced swelling and pain in the breasts may be exacerbated by a second effect, which is hypothesized to be caused by an insufficient synthesis of PGE 1. GLA-rich oils are prescribed to counteract the effects of prolactin on breast tissue by enhancing the production of series 1 anti-inflammatory prostaglandins.

9

Rediscovering Your Cycle And Your Body: The Three Primary Fertility Signs

You'll get a blank expression from the average woman if you mention that her body is a walking biological computer that contains the most insightful data regarding her fertility. Women of reproductive age can learn to recognize and record the three basic indications of fertility that their bodies produce with relative ease. With this information, individuals can learn a great deal about their cycle, the most evident of which being whether or not they can get pregnant today.

As you know, the three most common indications of ovulation that women produce are as follows:

1. Cervical fluid
2. Waking temperature
3. Cervical position

CERVICAL FLUID

In the beginning, you may notice a unique trend in the amount of cervical fluid that you produce. For many women, the first time they saw strange secretions coming out of their bodies at random times was "gross" and bewildering. They had no idea that these secretions had a purpose and followed a pattern until they learned to chart.

For most women, the second thing they may feel after learning about fertility symptoms is a sense of dissatisfaction and even anger at how little they had previously known about their own bodies. No, you didn't have recurrent vaginal infections on a regular basis. In fact, you weren't filthy or needed a wash to remove the "discharge." However, a great benefit of keeping a log of your cervical fluid is that you can distinguish between true vaginal infection and a symptomatic discharge. You should avoid using the "d-word" to describe your cervical fluid in the future. The term "discharge" is not used to describe men's healthy semen.

A woman's cervical fluid is like a man's seminal fluid. Every day, guys create seminal fluid because they are always fertile. A woman's fertility is limited to a few days around ovulation, and consequently, she produces the material that sperm need for sustenance and motility only during this time.

It's easy to understand. Sperm can only survive, migrate, and prosper in the presence of a medium. As soon as the sperm leave the penis, they need a comparable substance to keep them alive in the vagina. The only moment sperm survival is critical is when the egg is released. So, during each menstrual cycle, women-only generate a small amount of a substance that resembles semen.

Cervical fluid serves a variety of purposes. By creating an alkaline environment for sperm, an alkaline medium protects them from the acidic vaginal environment, one of its most important roles.

Cervical fluid in women begins to form and mimic seminal fluid in men in a pretty predictable way, to sum it up. As she nears ovulation, she notices an increase in spots. Remember that a woman's fluids grow more fertile as she nears ovulation. So, for example, her cervical fluid will have more fertile features following her menstruation and directly under the impact of increased estrogen. To illustrate how a woman's cervical fluid could change, check out The Continuum of Cervical Fluid: Sticky, Creamy, and Eggwhite. To be clear, they are merely a guide to assist you in discovering your own personal cycles.

Dry

Immediately following your period, you may get a dry vaginal sensation and notice nothing around the vaginal opening, which is common. It's possible that you'll feel a little bit of dampness, like if you were to touch your cheek for a split second. After a few seconds, the moisture on your finger would disappear.

That's how it usually feels like when there's no cervical fluid in the orifice. As estrogen levels begin to rise, you'll notice a "Point of Change" in your cycle, which indicates that you're nearing ovulation. After your menstruation has ended, you are likely to observe cervical fluid for the first time. It could happen on Day 6 for some people, and it could happen on Day 11 for others. It's critical to know how your own body responds to estrogen because every woman is unique.

Sticky

Cervical fluid is different for everyone, but the most important thing is that you'll notice it. Like the paste you used in elementary school, it may be gummy. It could also be flaky. There are times when it may even resemble the drying rubber cement, but the key thing is that it isn't truly wet at all. If identified before ovulation, this particular sort of cervical fluid, while not favorable to sperm survival, must be considered viable for contraceptive purposes.

Creamy

For the next few days, you may notice a wetter sort of cervical fluid. Creamy or lotion-like may be how some describe it. Just like hand lotion feels cool to the touch, it's possible that the vaginal opening will feel the same way. Even if it stretches to 3/8 of an inch, it will snap. Most importantly, this form of cervical fluid is wet, but it lacks the quality of the next and most fertile type of fluid yet. A transitional sort of secretion is one that lies between sticky and the most fertile and slippery qualities described next.

Eggwhite

In addition to resembling raw egg whites, the final and most viable cervical fluid is also the easiest to recognize. Stretches at least an inch and is either transparent or lubricative in nature (the ability to stretch is called spinnbarkeit, or spin for short). Make the phrase "stretchy, clear, or lubricative" your mantra. In addition, it may be streaked, yellow, pink or red in color, all of which indicate possible ovulation bleeding. It won't break if you stretch it. Your vagina will feel slippery even though you are unable to see anything. This is because of the lack of vision. Due to its high water content, it will often leave a circle of fluid on your underwear, as many of you have previously noticed.

Even if you can't see anything, your vaginal wetness and lubrication are vital indicators of high-quality cervical fluid. The slick nature of this extraordinarily fertile cervical fluid is once again its most crucial property. The lubricating vaginal sensation that normally goes along with it can last for a few days after the stretchy or clear cervical fluid has gone away. That tells you that you are still incredibly fertile. Sexual lubrication, on the other hand, should not be mistaken for vaginal sensations. Vaginal feeling is something you can feel or notice during wiping, but you don't have to pay attention to it to know what it is. When determining the fertility of cervical fluid, it is more necessary to focus on its quality than its quantity.

The cervical fluid changes rapidly when estrogen levels peak, often within a few hours. This is because estrogen levels drop suddenly, and progesterone levels rise just as the egg is about to be delivered. Non-fertilized cervical fluid generates a thick, sticky block that prevents the sperm from entering. As a result, the sperm that aren't trapped in the plug are also destroyed by the acidic vaginal environment.

Once the fertile-quality cervical fluid has formed for up to a week, it normally evaporates in less than a day. When the cervical fluid suddenly dries up, it is a good indicator that estrogen levels have dropped and progesterone has taken over. Most of the time, the absence of wet cervical fluid lasts for the entire cycle.

It is also possible for women to have a moist, egg-white-like sensation the day or two before menstruation. This may be linked to a decrease in progesterone that occurs before the uterine lining breaks down. As water flows out of the uterine lining, it causes the sensation of being very moist. Premature menstruation is not a sign of fertility because the egg will have been destroyed two weeks prior to this period.

One way to think about the changes in your cervical fluid is as a wave that slowly rises in height before crashing suddenly to the ground. The analogy holds even though hormones are less pronounced in humans than they are in animals.

Running tissue across your vaginal lips might assist you in identifying the true quality of the cervical fluid and vaginal sensation. Is there a lack of moisture that makes it difficult to move? Do you think it's going to be easy? Is it only gliding across? The tissue won't slide across your vaginal lips smoothly if you are dry or sticky. After ovulation, your cervical fluid becomes more viscous, making it easier for the tissue to move.

Knowing what's What

"The saddest example" I can think of is a woman I worked with years ago who didn't understand what normal cervical fluid was like.

After taking the pill for six years, Joan came to my class for the first time. Before attending my class, she had to suffer a diagnostic test that she didn't need because she didn't know how to interpret the fascinating signals her body sends throughout each cycle.

When Joan had a bowel movement, she would occasionally see a slick material on the toilet paper. Due to the frequency and timing of her bathroom visits, she grew very anxious that something was wrong with her digestive system. Colonoscopy was recommended to rule out inflammatory bowel illness or polyps, according to the doctor. Why is this the case?

The fertilized egg white was oozing from Joan's vagina, which was completely normal and frequent. Tissue paper can be used to disseminate this type because it is so slick and abundant. Since she generated egg whites exclusively during ovulation, she must have observed this slippery stuff from time to time.

This does not imply, however, that routine colonoscopies are not necessary. Starting at 50, you should obtain one every five to ten years as part of your proactive approach to health. However, I have a feeling that if you're reading this, you're not quite that old. If you were taught the ins and outs of slippery cervical fluid, you would know to look for signs of it, especially when bearing down on the toilet.

For me, hearing about women like Brandy, who have undergone pointless and stressful testing, is one of the most motivating reasons to spread awareness about their own bodies' natural cues regarding their reproductive health. That doesn't mean, however, that women don't experience genuine infections or other health issues. Simply put, women should be educated on what is considered normal in order to better recognize abnormal behavior in themselves. Cervical fluid can be masked by a variety of causes, including, but not limited to:

- Douching
- Vaginal infections
- Seminal fluid
- Arousal fluid
- Spermicides and lubricants
- Antihistamines (which can dry it)

A sticky, rubber cement or wet type of discharge that persists for weeks or longer may indicate cervicitis or cervical erosion. For the sake of your cervical fluid, you should address both of these illnesses, even if they're not life-threatening.

It's common for women to wonder whether or not the cervical fluid is the same as seminals or arousal liquid. Cervical fluid, on the other hand, remains on your finger until you wash it off, but the other two are much thinner and dry faster.

In the event that one of the three symptoms is unclear, you may rest assured that you can cross-check the other two to be sure you have a correct interpretation of your fertility.

WAKING (BASAL BODY) TEMPERATURE

The waking temperature is perhaps the simplest symptom to detect because it is usually extremely graphic and objective. A fun task for many women who have been tracking their fertility for a few months is to forecast when their temps will change. For pre-and postovulatory temps, a woman's waking temperature ranges from 97.0 to 97.7 degrees F, respectively. After ovulation, they tend to remain elevated for 12 to 16 days until her next menstruation. While pregnant, her levels would remain elevated for most of her pregnancy, with a modest decrease a few months before delivery.

Progesterone, a heat-inducing hormone, is responsible for the spike in temperature that occurs within a day or two of ovulation. The corpus luteum is the source of progesterone. Ovulation has already occurred; therefore, a rise in temperature is usually a clue that it has.

You'll need to practice "seeing the forest through the trees" when analyzing temperatures. Find a pattern of lows and highs if you want to succeed at this task. Your pre-ovulation and post-ovulation temps will fluctuate in a narrow range, while your pre-ovulation and post-ovulation temps will fluctuate in a wider range. The key is to look at the big picture rather than getting caught up in the minutiae of the day-to-day.

When I first taught at a women's clinic years ago, I saw how useful this approach was. Clients began calling me within a few weeks of the first lesson, convinced that they weren't ovulating. In the Paleolithic Age, before e-mail, when people read me their temperatures over the phone, the trend was clear. Seeing what I saw, I had no idea why they couldn't see it either. That's when it hit me. Instead of perceiving the pattern, they were focused on the fact that it went up and down, then back up, again and over again. Stand back and take a look at the big picture. You may want to chart many cycles before relying on FAM as a form of birth control if you find that your temperatures aren't clearly visible.

Estrogen lowers pre-ovulatory temperatures, while heat-inducing progesterone raises post-ovulatory temperatures.

Progestation is a good way to recall the second part of the cycle as the "progesterone" phase, as the hormone is also known. If you think of it as a human incubator for an egg that recently hatched, then this is the part of the cycle where the temperature rises.

Again, a spike in waking temperatures nearly invariably means that ovulation has already occurred. As with the cervical fluid and cervical position, it does not indicate impending ovulation. You should also be aware that only a small percentage of cycles will see women ovulation when their temperature is at its lowest point. When it comes to fertility, women should not rely on a pre-ovulatory temperature decrease. Instead, they should monitor the cervical fluid and cervical posture for signs of impending ovulation.

There are a few things to be on the lookout for that could raise your waking temperature:

- Taking it if you have a fever, drank alcohol the night before, or slept for less than three hours straight or at a period that is significantly different from the norm
- Using a heating pad or electric blanket when you wouldn't ordinarily

In the following chapter, you'll learn that you don't have to worry about fluctuating temperatures. This is due to the fact that they can be ignored without affecting the method's precision. However, two additional daily signals are provided by FAM to double-check your fertility.

Temps, Stress, and the Dreaded Late Period

When it comes to figuring out how long your cycle will be, waking temps can be highly helpful because they can tell if you've had an ovulation delay, which can cause your cycle to be longer than typical. If the weather warms up, you should expect your period to arrive between 12 and 16 days later. You'll be able to pinpoint your precise postovulatory range after charting for a few cycles. (As previously mentioned, the phase following ovulation does not differ significantly for the majority of women.)

During one of her cycles, when she was moving from one house to another, one of my clients reported classic delayed ovulation. There were three things going on in my life at the time that could have delayed ovulation.

As a 31-year-old woman, her cycles ranged from approximately 26 to 32 days. She had all the indicators that she was nearing ovulation in November. In addition to her cervix rising and growing more open and soft, the cervical fluid in her was becoming moist. After 16 days, she had to wash her walls and transfer her belongings out of the apartment she'd been living in and into her new house, which meant she had to wash and relocate every box she had. It was also necessary for her to talk at the nearby midwifery school before boarding a jet at rush hour to deliver the same lecture at another conference in another state the following morning. So what happened? She was in a constant state of flux, juggling work, family, and personal obligations. Everything about her said, "Tell you what. As long as you're ready, I'll put your ovulation on wait." Even though she didn't ovulate until Day 24, she had a 38-day cycle because of it! She might have thought she was pregnant if she hadn't been charting, as she'd never before had such a long period of time in her cycle.

An important lesson can be learned from this scenario. It's common for women who don't chart to worry about their periods being late since they don't realize that long cycles are usually due to ovulating later, which is easily spotted through waking temperatures.

To illustrate my argument that ovulation can be delayed or even prevented by stress, travel, relocating, illness, medicine, hard exercise and a sudden weight shift, I utilized the experience of this client. However, if you keep a log of your temperature readings, you'll be able to tell when your ovulation may be delayed. Knowing this knowledge can save you a lot of stress and uncertainty, regardless of whether you're attempting to avoid or achieve pregnancy.

CERVICAL POSITION (OPTIONAL SIGN)

Intercourse can be uncomfortable in some postures, haven't you noticed? It's possible that you have fond memories of a quiet Sunday morning with your significant other. When you awoke the next morning, you were overcome with desire for him and slid on top of him. Even though you were eager to revisit that great day just one week later, you were surprised to find yourself filled with sharp anguish instead. The situation puzzled me. This time, why is it so difficult?

Then there are those times when it appears impossible to find the cervix to implant your diaphragm or cervical cap, and those times when it is relatively simple. A more serious issue is that there may appear to be no room at all for it. Have you ever been told by a doctor that you appeared to be pregnant during a pelvic exam, despite the fact that she had only inserted a speculum?

Cervix, the region of the uterus closest to the vaginal opening, goes through an array of intriguing changes during the course of your menstrual cycle, all of which are plainly detectable. At your fingertips, the cervix can provide a plethora of information about your fertility. Every cycle, the cervix transforms into a perfect "biological gate" through which the sperm can pass on their journey to the egg, much like a cervical fluid does. As the uterus softens and the fallopian tubes become more permeable, the sperm can easily travel through. Due to estrogen's action on the uterine ligaments, the cervix elevates as well.

Once you've had your period, your cervix will begin to change as a direct result of estrogen. The acronym SHOW is a simple method to recall how your cervix feels as you approach ovulation, as illustrated in the graphic below.

CERVICAL POSITION CHANGES DURING THE CYCLE

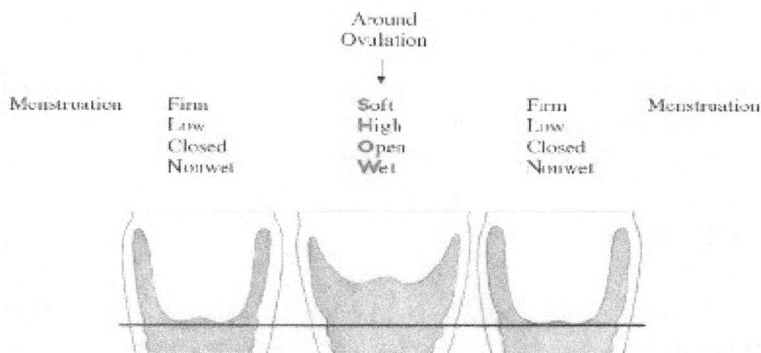

Menstruation	Firm	Around Ovulation ↓ Soft	Firm	Menstruation
	Low	High	Low	
	Closed	Open	Closed	
	Nonwet	Wet	Nonwet	

Let's go over each of these aspects one by one. If your cervix is like the tip of your nose, it's usually solid. Only when you're getting close to ovulation does it become soft and mushy. When estrogen levels are very high around ovulation, the cervix rises and opens, giving the appearance of a dimple. Finally, when the egg is going to be delivered, the cervix itself generates fertile-quality wet cervical fluid.

SECONDARY FERTILITY SIGNS

It is fortunate for many women that they are able to see other indicators on a regular basis, all of which assist them to better understand their cycles. These are known as secondary fertility markers because they don't occur in every woman or every cycle. However, they are still quite beneficial in helping women pinpoint their fertile and infertile periods.

In the days leading up to ovulation, secondary indications may include:

- Ovulatory spotting
- Pain or achiness near the ovaries
- Fuller vaginal lips or swollen vulva
- Swollen lymph gland
- Increased sexual feelings
- Abdominal bloating
- Water retention
- Increased energy level
- Heightened sense of vision, smell, and taste
- Increased sensitivity in breasts and skin
- Breast tenderness

An abrupt drop in estrogen soon before ovulation is thought to cause the first symptom on the list above, ovulatory spotting. The lining may leak a tiny amount of blood until the progesterone takes over because it has not yet been released to sustain it. As far as spotting goes, it can come in any shade, from hardly noticeable to blazing red, and it's more common in women who have extended cycles.

It's not uncommon for women to confuse different types of bleeding, and Britney was no exception. She contacted to inquire about the possibility of using FAM as a form of birth control but was concerned that her "very short cycles" precluded her from being a good candidate. "Literally every two weeks, but alternating heavy, light, heavy, light," she remarked when I inquired about them. She was most likely going through a usual long cycle with classic ovulatory spotting. So, I urged her to sign up for my Fertility Awareness class that I teach. Even if she doesn't use FAM for contraception anymore, she has a greater understanding of her own body than she did previously.

There are a number of hypotheses as to why women have aches and pains during their pregnancies. These symptoms can occur before, during, or after your ovulation, and it's impossible to tell for sure which time period.

- **Dull achiness:** To explain this, it's believed that as eggs compete for dominance in the ovaries, they're swollen. Since both ovaries swell with developing follicles as the woman approaches ovulation, it's usually felt as a widespread aching in the abdomen.
- **A sharp pain:** Only one side of the ovarian wall can be felt for a brief period of time after the egg has passed through the wall.
- **Crampiness:** Blood or follicular fluid leakage from an egg follicle that has ruptured is most likely to blame for causing discomfort to the stomach lining in this case. Ovulation contractions in the fallopian tubes may possibly be to blame for this.

Because there are so many possible pains, none of them can be relied upon as a sole indicator of fertility. Aside from the three basic indications, ovulatory discomfort is a good secondary fertility indicator. Many women experience mittelschmerz (middle pain) around the time of ovulation. It can last anywhere from a few minutes to a few hours, and it usually happens on the side of the body where ovulation takes place the most frequently.

Swollen vulva is an interesting secondary fertility indicator that can be seen right before ovulation. Some women's vulvae get puffier on one side when their cervical fluid becomes more slippery and moist (the side on which they are ovulating). Additionally, another secondary fertility indicator is noteworthy since it can help you decide which side of the uterus will ovulate.

You may notice a little lymph gland grow to the size of a pea as you approach ovulation if you pay attention. You can feel the lymph node sign by lying down and placing your palm near your groin, as shown in the figure below. Your index finger may be able to detect the lymph gland's tenderness and expanded size by placing your middle finger slightly above the pulsating artery. Ovulation is more likely to occur on this side. Charting isn't required, but it's fun to have another indicator to keep an eye on.

Checking the lymph node as you approach ovulation

In addition to the indicators described above, you may discover other secondary fertility signs by charting. As a counselor, I've dealt with a wide range of issues:

Ovulation-related hiccups occur for Mary. Every cycle, around the time of ovulation, the skin on Anna's thumb develops a painful lesion. It wasn't until she learned to chart that she discovered what was causing the problem. Ovulation is a time when Jessie's sense of smell is so enhanced that she can smell her chef-cooking husband's for days following, and wide windows don't help alleviate nausea she suffers. When she eats something containing mustard, even though she washes her hands thoroughly afterward, she can still smell it! The onion-garlic dish she can make while she isn't in her reproductive phase has no effect on her.

Women are often taken aback when they realize that all of this occurs on a regular basis inside their bodies. In the fifth grade, all they learned about menstruation was whether to use tampons or sanitary napkins.

10

How To Track Your Fertility Signs With A Chart

It's true: keeping track of your fertile days will help you become pregnant more often. Or perhaps assist you in figuring out which days to forgo intercourse in order to avoid getting pregnant?

Keeping track of the days when you're most fertile (a practice known as "fertility awareness") might be beneficial whether you're just starting your journey to parenthood or have been trying for some time without success. Predicting when ovulation will occur is as simple as getting to know your body and its natural cycle.

Tracking your fertility can be done in a variety of ways, including applications and devices. Certain techniques work better when combined with others, and some are more effective when used alone. To help you find the optimal fertility awareness method for your body, we've broken down each method. Getting pregnant (or not) is made a whole lot easier with our picks for the best fertility tracking apps and tools.

What Is Fertility Awareness?

Awareness of your menstrual cycle's viable window (also known as ovulation tracking, ovulation tracking, natural family planning, or fertility charting) is an important part of fertility awareness. Your ovaries release an egg every month on the day of ovulation, and this viable window includes the five days before and after that time. Based on the theory that sperm can survive in the uterus for up to five days and an egg can survive for 12-24 hours after ovulation, these are the six days when you're most likely to become pregnant.

Approaches for determining when your body is entering the fertile window are known as fertility awareness-based methods (FABMs). FABMs can be used as a natural form of birth control, letting you know which days of the month to avoid sexual activity or using a barrier method like a condom in order to predict when you're most likely to become pregnant.

Contrary to popular belief, using FABMs to prevent pregnancy is not as effective as other methods of birth control, such as pills or an IUD.)

BENEFITS OF TRACKING FERTILITY

FABMs can assist in eliminating the element of surprise associated with ovulation timing, given that there are only six fertile days in each month. In a typical 28-day menstrual cycle, your fertile window is believed to be between days 10 and 17, according to clinical guidelines. However, according to 2000 research, 70% of women ovulated outside of this time window. The day of ovulation for women with regular cycles was shown to be very variable, according to the same study. Adding to this, a study published in 2006 indicated that factors including stress, food, and sleep could alter your cycle duration and ovulation.

FABMs come into play here. Throughout your menstrual cycle, your body sends forth signals regarding your fertility. The sooner you understand what to look for and how to keep track of these indications, the sooner you'll be able to discover your own unique pattern.

FABMs can accurately predict your fertile window by as much as 76-88 percent when used correctly. Checking and charting your fertility indicators every day and consulting with a health care practitioner who knows how to do it properly is essential for the best results. FABMs are most effective when used with a range of other methods. Tracking your fertility can help you in the following ways.

1. Natural and healthy family planning.

Your odds of having a baby can be improved upon. When trying to figure out when you're most fertile, keeping track of your ovulation cycle can be quite beneficial. Because each woman's ovulation cycle is distinct, no two are exactly alike. Monthly fluctuations are also possible. You can better plan your pregnancy if you understand your cycle and know when you'll be able to conceive naturally.

2. Avoid unplanned pregnancy

Contraception is not 100% effective, and some of the ones don't work as well as they should. Some tablets have a failure rate of 7 percent, whereas condoms have a failure rate of 16 percent. You're taking a risk when you play at this level. To avoid an unplanned pregnancy, it's important to make it a daily ritual to verify your ovulation.

3. Your general health.

Any anomalies can be discovered earlier. It's especially important for newly sexually mature ladies. It is feasible to detect warning signals of an issue before it becomes life-threatening for the patient.

4. Schedule activities around your ovulation

Research has shown that ovulating women experience and behave differently than non-ovulating women due to hormonal shifts. You'll undoubtedly want to use your ovulation cycle to help you plan some significant activities, such as business meetings or vacations. Keeping tabs on your ovulation cycle is a smart idea.

5. Understand and control your body

Another advantage of keeping track of your ovulation is that you will gain a better understanding of your own body and how it works. Knowing your body's needs can save you from using medications that aren't necessary and putting yourself through excessive stress.

Tracking ovulation can help avoid an ectopic pregnancy, as well. If you're over 40 and keep track of your ovulation cycle on a regular basis, you'll know when you're pregnant and can make an appointment with your doctor. He or she will then begin to supervise your treatment from the early stage of pregnancy, discover any anomalies and shift any eggs growing halfway in your fallopian tubes. He or she. One percent of women over the age of 40 have had an ectopic pregnancy fertility issue, according to a poll.

FERTILITY AWARENESS: BEST METHODS YOU CAN USE TO TRACK YOUR FERTILE DAYS

Calendar Method (Standard Days Method)

Your menstrual cycle's length and the date of your last period are used to determine when you are most likely to ovulate with this procedure. It is assumed that the typical menstrual cycle is between 21 and 35 days long and that the average luteal phase is 14 days. It's called the luteal phase because it occurs between the day of ovulation and the first day of your period. Your luteal phase, like the length of your menstrual cycle, can range from 10 to 15 days.

Menstrual cycles should be tracked for at least six cycles in order to obtain a good idea of how long your average cycle is. Your luteal phase (if you don't know it, use 14 days) and your last period's start date can be used to determine when your fertile window is most likely to fall on a paper calendar or an online calendar or app.

As a result of its heavy reliance on averages, this approach isn't always 100 percent reliable. Even if you have fairly regular periods and have been charting your cycle for some time, your cycle and ovulation date may fluctuate from cycle to month. Those with more irregular cycles should figure out their average cycle length and then allow themselves a longer fertile window than the standard six days to accommodate for any calendar charting errors.

Basal Body Temperature Method

When you first wake up in the morning, your basal body temperature (BBT) is the temperature within your body. As your cycle progresses, your basal body temperature (BBT) rises and falls, with a low point just prior to ovulation and a high point just after ovulation. During ovulation, progesterone levels rise, resulting in a rise in temperature. You can discover ovulation signals by taking your BBT every morning before you get out of bed.

During the two weeks following ovulation, your BBT will remain elevated before dropping again before your next period. It's a good sign that ovulation has occurred if the temperature rises for at least three days.

Charting your BBT for at least three months is suggested in order to accurately forecast your reproductive window.

Cervical Mucus Method

Glands in and around your cervix produce cervical mucus (vaginal discharge), which has two functions:

1. To keep things out of your uterus outside of your fertile window;
2. To nourish and transport sperm into your uterus while you are fertile.

You can use the cervical mucus method (also known as the Billing Ovulation Method) as a way to determine when you're going to ovulate by monitoring the color, texture, and volume of your cervical mucus. In general, less fertile women tend to have a dryer, stickier cervical mucus, whereas more fertile women tend to have wetter, thinner mucus. After ovulation, your cervical mucus will begin to thin to the point where it resembles the consistency of raw egg white. This increases the alkalinity of the sperm's surroundings and makes it easier for them to pass through the cervix.

Menstrual cycle: Your cervical mucus goes through these stages:

- Ovulating – Mucus is drier or more viscous than normal
- Mucus is creamy, which indicates that ovulation is imminent.
- The mucus is wet and runny, indicating that ovulation is imminent.
- Wet, stretchy mucus that looks like raw egg whites indicates ovulation has happened.

Unless you are on your period, you should check your mucus every day and record the results on a chart when using this method to establish your fertile window. You might be a little apprehensive about this, but remember that it's natural and your body's way of preparing you for pregnancy. Because it's difficult to tell the differences in mucus consistency without a doctor's advice, you should start using this procedure with their guidance. The color of your cervical mucus can vary if you take medicine, use feminine hygiene products, douch, engage in sexual intercourse, breastfeed, or have a pelvic exam in which lubrication is employed.

It is most accurate when used in conjunction with the BBT technique. Cervical mucus is 97 percent accurate when used alone, according to the Centers for Disease Control and Prevention

The symptothermal Method

Combining the BBT, cervical mucus, and calendar approaches, we have the Symptothermal Method (STM). The overall efficacy of these three approaches is 99.6 percent.

Each of the three ways uses various signals to anticipate your fertile window, making the STM the most accurate method for raising your awareness of your fertile window. When your temperature or cervical mucus is out of wack due to stress or illness, this helps you to narrow down your fertile days and provides you with reliable backup methods.

Cervical Position Method

A woman's cervix undergoes numerous changes during her menstrual cycle. In order to identify if you're in your fertile window, you can look at your cervical position, which consists of these three physical traits.

Your cervix is lower in your vagina and stiffer during the start of your menstrual cycle. You'll notice that your cervix begins to soften as you get closer to ovulation.

Preparing for ovulation can be easier when you know when your cervical position is at its most fertile.

Ovulation Predicator Kits

In terms of accuracy, ovulation prediction kits are up there with the best. Colors on ovulation test strips indicate when your luteinizing hormone (LH) levels are rising, just like pregnancy urine tests. An increase in LH levels normally suggests that ovulation will take place within 12 to 36 hours after the onset of the rise in LH levels.

To accurately identify an LH spike, you may need to perform the test numerous times daily over several days. Ovulation can be predicted 80 percent of the time using a five-day cycle of using a test strip. If you test for 10 days in a row, your success rate rises to 95%. If you are trying to get pregnant, it is recommended that you have sex every day for the next two to three days after ovulation has been anticipated.

Saliva Ferning Tests

Did you know saliva may tell you when you're about to ovulate? When saliva is dried, fern-like crystals (from where the term ferning is from) are formed, which is why it's known as a fertile window. A drop of saliva is placed on a lens included in saliva ferning kits. If the unique fern-like crystals are not visible after five minutes, use the accompanying viewing scope.

Within 24 to 72 hours of the first crystal forms being discovered, ovulation is likely to occur. Ovatel® and the Fertile-Focus® Saliva Ovulation Microscope are examples of saliva ferning tests.

11

Anovulation And Irregular Cycles

No one here is a Barbie. As much as the fashion industry would like us to believe that women should all be 5'9" and model slim, the truth is that women come in many shapes and sizes. The old wives' tale that all women have 28-day cycles and ovulate on Day 14 is just wrong, as you should know by now.

The length of a woman's menstrual cycle might vary not only from month to month but it also depends on the stage of life in which she is. In some situations, such as adolescence, the discontinuation of the pill, nursing, or the onset of menopause, you may only have sporadic ovulation for several months at a time. Temporary conditions, including illness, travel, anxiety, or exercise, might potentially affect your cycle.

What's great about keeping track of your menstrual cycles is that you'll be able to better manage and comprehend your body's everyday processes, no matter what your life circumstances are. So, what are the characteristics of a cycle that is not regular? Cycles that fall within the range of 21 to 35 days are considered normal unless there are additional signs and symptoms that indicate something is wrong. If they fall outside of that range or are accompanied by inconsistent amounts of bleeding, you should consult your doctor. In general, the quality of menstruation after ovulation is quite consistent, so if your cycles are erratic, with bleeding that can be light or heavy or red or brown or even without clots or clots, it's generally an indication that you are not ovulating normally, if at all.

Depending on your reproductive status, you may notice a shift in how your indicators are displayed over time.

- A typical cycle: In a typical cycle, your body gets ready for the egg release in a predictable and timely manner. After your period, estrogen levels rise, and you'll experience a few days of potentially no or sticky cervical fluid, followed by a few days of steadily wetter and more fertile-quality fluid. Following egg release, your cervical fluid will quickly dry up until the cycle begins again.
- An anovulatory phase (low body weight, breastfeeding, pre-menopause, etc.): This is a term used to describe the times when ovulation takes longer for women. Your body might possibly take as long as a year or more to build up enough estrogen to ovulate in these unusual conditions. Many failed attempts at ovulation may be necessary before your body is eventually able to ovulate successfully. You may observe "patches" of cervical fluid during this period. Wet areas may be interspersed with dry ones rather than the typical accumulation seen in normal cycles.

This chapter focuses on what happens in your body when you don't ovulate or ovulate very infrequently.

DIFFERENT PHASES OF ANOVULATION OR IRREGULAR CYCLES IN WOMEN'S LIVES

Adolescence

Between the ages of 12 and 14, most American girls begin their menstrual cycle. When periods begin, it does not necessarily guarantee that an egg will be released. Because estrogen levels fluctuate, menstrual cycles in teenage girls tend to be unpredictable because they don't always begin at the same time each month. As the hormonal feedback system matures, the process can take several years. Adolescent menstrual periods can therefore be quite variable, with numerous anovulatory cycles scattered throughout.

Coming off of the Pill

Women's displeasure with the myriad side effects, both subtle and overt, they typically encounter while on the pill is one of the most compelling reasons for them to learn about FAM. It's breakthrough bleeding if you don't have headaches or weight gain. However, my main concern as a women's health educator is that women are administered the pill to "control" their menstrual cycles.

As a result, their cycles frequently return to normal after they stop taking the pill. This is a major drawback of this method of treatment. A woman may be shocked to discover, ten years after taking the pill to regulate her cycles at the age of 23, that her cycles have returned to their pre-pill irregularity, and she has a condition such as PCOS that was never treated when its symptoms were first revealed when she decides to try to get pregnant at the age of 33. Before using the pill, I believe women should be informed about the pill's potentially harmful side effects, including the potential for fertility concerns to be masked by the pill.

Pregnancy and Breastfeeding

As a result of being pregnant or breastfeeding, many women prefer that their periods have ceased. After conception, a woman's body is incapable of conceiving again. Of course, this is rational. Pregnant women do not ovulate until after the birth of their child. She may not ovulate again for months or even years following the birth of her child if she breastfeeds "on-demand," which means that she feeds the baby whenever he or she cries. It's because prolactin, a hormone that lowers FSH and LH, is stimulated every time a baby sucks, which directly affects ovulation. A breastfed baby must suckle continuously throughout the day and night in order for breastfeeding to be effective in preventing egg release.

Every day, regardless of whether it is dry, sticky, or a combination of the three, a breastfeeding woman will experience the same Basic Infertile Pattern (BIP). Because of the low estrogen levels, which are indirectly caused by the hormone prolactin, fertile-quality cervical fluid will not be produced at the beginning of her pregnancy. Be aware of the Point of Change in cervical fluid quality that suggests that ovulation is about to begin again for breastfeeding women.

Pre-menopause

Menopause occurs when a woman's menstrual cycle is no longer regular. It usually occurs at about 51 years of age. Even though menopause can take as long as 10 years, fertility actually begins to decline about 13 years before the final period. Premenopausal women may notice that their menstrual periods begin to seem different than they have in the past. Due to shortened luteal stages, cycle lengths initially decrease. But when the number of times an egg is released decreases, the cycles will become longer and longer until they reach a maximum. Finally, there are no more cycles. It is widely accepted that a woman has entered menopause when she has gone a year without having a period.

THE DIFFERENCE BETWEEN AN ANOVULATORY CYCLE AND BEING ANOVULATORY

Most women experience an "anovulatory cycle" from time to time throughout their lives. Your ovulation may have been delayed because of a fever that arose just before you were ready to ovulate. It's possible that you've tried a truly crazy diet of cotton balls (no joke—some have!), which effectively informed your body it was full but that until you get your act together, ovulation won't happen. You may have gone on a seven-week vacation to Vladivostok and not ovulated again until you returned.

On the other hand, "being anovulatory" refers to a condition that can linger for weeks or even months until it is resolved. Breastfeeding, being underweight, or having a medical condition like PCOS or hypothyroidism can all cause this.

AN OVULATORY RIDDLE FOR YOUR CYCLE-SAVVY FRIENDS

Is there a difference between an ovulatory cycle without menstruation and a menstruating cycle without ovulation? Think about it for a time before moving on.

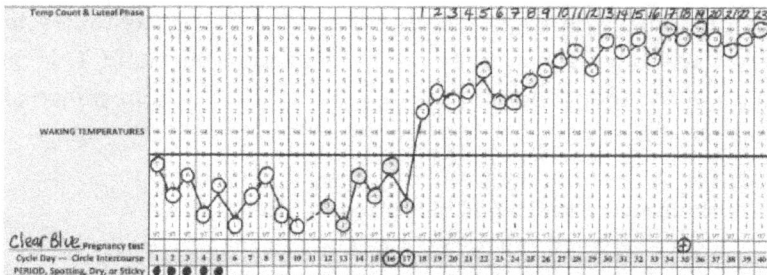

Jennifer's chart. Pregnant women typically experience this type of temperature pattern. By the next morning's temperature change, it is almost certain that Jennifer had ovulated on Day 17. There are over 18 high temps on her chart since the shift, which indicates she's pregnant.

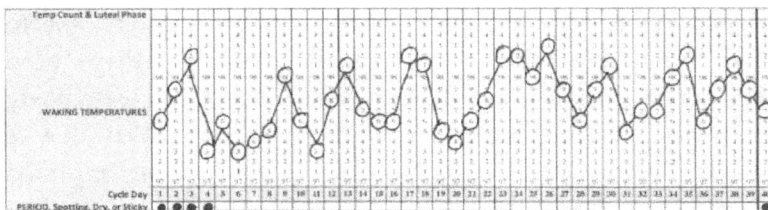

Kate's chart. An example of a normal temperature pattern during an anovulatory period of pregnancy. Anovulatory bleeding, which is not menstruation, is what Kate experienced after she didn't have a temperature shift indicating ovulation on Day 40.

Pregnant women in the first scenario are virtually always found in the latter. An anovulatory cycle occurred in this case. On paper, the two possibilities appear extremely different.

ANOTHER GREAT REASON TO CHART

Non-charting women who are in anovulatory cycles may mistakenly believe they are menstruation properly. If ovulation has not occurred, why would they continue to have bleeding? During this type of bleeding, the uterine lining continues to grow without reaching the essential ovulation threshold. One or both of the following may occur, resulting in the appearance of menstruation:

- "Estrogen withdrawal hemorrhage" occurs when estrogen levels fall below a certain threshold.

- It's more normal for the endometrium to build up slowly over a protracted period of time, eventually reaching a point where it can no longer support itself. The uterine lining is discharged in "estrogen breakthrough bleeding" because it lacks progesterone.

It's possible to think you're just menstruating in both cases, but the sort of bleeding could be different if you weren't charting. It is possible for the flow to be abnormally light or heavy, and the timing can lead to cycle lengths that are all over the map.

COMMON CAUSES OF TEMPORARY ANOVULATION OR IRREGULAR CYCLES

Other prevalent causes of women's inability to ovulate, whether short-term or long-term, include the following:

Illness

It's possible that getting sick will have no effect on your cycle, but if it does, the severity of the effect depends on the stage of the cycle you're in at the time. Your ovulation may be delayed or perhaps prevented if your illness arises before that time. Because the luteal phase has a continuous life span of 12 to 16 days that is not impacted by circumstances such as sickness, travel, or exercise, it is unlikely to have an impact on your cycle if it happens afterward. The length of the luteal phase is even more regular for each individual woman, and it will seldom vary by more than a day or two.

Regardless, it is at times like these that examining your cervix and other secondary markers of fertility can help you establish if your fever had no influence or if it had an impact but delayed or prevented ovulation. Using FAM as a form of birth control when the circumstances are ambiguous requires utmost care.

Ovarian Cysts

Temporary anovulation and irregular cycles are frequently caused by this. If you don't ovulate as a result of them, the most likely culprit is a cyst that formed early in your cycle. It's possible that they'll show up in the second part of your cycle if they lead you to have irregular periods. In either case, they're not likely to be life-threatening.

Travel

Traveling has a tendency to mess with your cycle. While some women are lucky enough to have periods that come and go according to plan even while they are away from home, others must deal with the uncertainty of not knowing whether or not they will get their period at all. Relaxation is still stressful to your body despite how enjoyable a vacation may be. Delaying ovulation can cause protracted periods of infertility in many women. Some women completely stop ovulating and receiving their periods.

Again, monitoring your cycle can be quite beneficial in figuring out what's going on with your body.. and what's not. It's important to remember, though, that traveling is a period when it's especially essential to chart all three signs to comprehend any misunderstandings that come from the interruption in your life. In particular, keep an eye out for anything that could impact your temperature.

Exercise

The ovulation cycle can be slowed or even halted entirely if you engage in strenuous exercise. There is a chance that you will use this as an excuse not to work out. Those who are competitive athletes with low body fat to total body weight ratios appear to be the most susceptible. Most at risk are female athletes like marathon runners and swimmers, as well as gymnasts and dancers in various forms of classical ballet. Athletes appear to be unable to distinguish between physical and emotional stress, food, and even variations in thyroid metabolism when it comes to fat ratio. A woman's cycle can be affected by any or all of these factors.

Weight Gain or Loss

Obesity is necessary for a healthy ovulatory cycle in most women; hence a BMI of 20-24, or 22% body fat, is recommended. Calculating your BMI is as simple as looking at a chart online. As a result of their extreme thinness, many women with anorexia have no menstrual cycle at all. As a result, they don't create the hormones required for ovulation. It's possible that women may stop menstruating if they drop 10 to 15 percent of their total body weight (or around one-third of their body fat). The combination of lean body fat and the stress of competition can cause female athletes to stop menstruation.

A French couple who had been trying to conceive for five years was one of my customers. Because he was a doctor, he feared the class would be too basic for them, so he requested a one-on-one meeting instead. As soon as they walked into my office, I knew something was wrong. A tall, slender woman, she stood out among the crowd. Despite my best efforts to persuade her otherwise, she flatly refused to eat any fat, even when I suggested it would help with her periods. They both insisted, though, that they couldn't understand why she wasn't conceiving, given how well she cared for herself. In fact, she said she hadn't had a period in five years when I pressed her for an explanation of her menstrual cycles.

I was shocked. Despite the fact that she wasn't menstrual, she was unable to conceive, despite the fact that she was educated and a physician. I was perplexed as to why they believed she was fertile when she hadn't had a period for so long! Their response left me speechless. Her doctor had once inquired about her method of birth control during a previous attempt to avoid pregnancy. Because she wasn't menstruating, they didn't utilize birth control, she explained. At the time, her doctor advised her to take precautions regardless because she may still ovulate at any time. That one remark that she may ovulate at any time convinced her that she was actually fertile.

If the couple's objective is to have children, the odds of pregnancy must be viewed differently. Her doctor was correct in terms of contraception; women must protect themselves because ovulation occurs before menstruation every time. A lady who is attempting to get pregnant and does not menstruate certainly does not have ovulation. It's easy to confuse the risk of unintended pregnancy with the chance of a pregnancy that is desired. Because they left for France shortly after we met, I'll never know what happened to them, but I can only presume that they dealt with her anovulatory problem.

Women who are obese are at the other extreme of the range. Their cycles may also come to an end. There's a good chance that you're thinking, "Wait a minute. Earlier, she indicated it could be an issue if the lady is too thin; today, she says the same thing could be a problem if she is too overweight." It's just the way women's bodies are! When there is too much fat tissue, the hormonal feedback loop that signals the maturation of egg follicles is disrupted.

Stress

Stress, both physiological and psychological, is a leading suspect in the development of unusually protracted cycles. When stress enters a cycle, it tends to slow down rather than speed up ovulation. As you may be aware, the length of a cycle is determined by the time at which ovulation happens; the later it occurs, the longer the cycle will be. Stress can actually prevent ovulation from occurring at all if it is severe enough.

MEDICAL CAUSES OF ANOVULATION OR IRREGULAR CYCLES

Many other medical conditions can lead women to stop ovulating for good, such as those listed above. These diseases are treatable, but you'll need to contact a doctor to find out what's causing your irregular periods or anovulation.

The sooner you see a doctor, regardless of whether or not you're trying to conceive, the better. There may be a medical disease affecting women with irregular menstrual cycles, not only because of the impact on their general health but also because of the impact on fertility. If you're attempting to avoid conception, a medical issue may make the Fertility Awareness Method more difficult to employ. In addition, it can thwart your efforts to get pregnant. If you experience any of the following signs or symptoms, you should schedule an appointment with your physician to have a full physical examination.

Hypothyroidism

If you're experiencing an anovulatory cycle, one of the first things you should look into is the condition of your thyroid gland, which is the bow-shaped gland located at the base of your neck.

Polycystic Ovarian Syndrome (PCOS)

Chances are, even if you've never heard of it, you know someone who does or has been affected by it in some manner. About 10% of women have PCOS, which is one of the most prevalent underlying reasons for anovulation and irregular menstrual cycles. This deadly hormone imbalance affects almost every organ in the body. There is a clear message here: consult a doctor (ideally a reproductive endocrinologist) as soon as possible if your cycles are extremely irregular, if they go more than 35 days, or you don't seem to ovulate at all.

Endometriosis

In women with this condition, the uterine lining implants outside the uterus, resulting in a wide range of symptoms. In the same way as PCOS, it is a pretty common problem. Not to the extent that PCOS causes irregular cycles.

Excessive Prolactin (Hyperprolactinaemia)

Because it circulates in nursing women and is often partly responsible for suppressing ovulation in women who are fully breastfeeding, prolactin is commonly referred to as the breastfeeding hormone. In rare cases, a woman who hasn't given birth or isn't breastfeeding may have a hormone level in her body that prevents ovulation from occurring at all. Pituitary tumors may be to blame for this. Regardless, it's a problem that may be treated fairly quickly and effectively.

Primary Ovarian Insufficiency (POI)

Premature Menopause (PM) and Premature Ovarian Failure (POF) are still terms used to describe this illness. However, it's true that the ovaries may stop working regularly before the age of 40 and, in rare cases, even earlier in the teen years. The ovaries don't always stop working, so women may continue to menstruate intermittently even though their cycles will be erratic and finally stop.

However, perimenopause-like symptoms, including irregular periods, hot flashes, and vaginal dryness, may also occur as a result of decreased estrogen production in POI. Women may also experience discomfort during intercourse as a result of the thinned vaginal walls.

Women with this illness have two main concerns:

1. POI is a major endocrine condition that has to be addressed. After the age of 51, women with POI should consider taking estrogen-progestin therapy to help prevent osteoporosis and possibly heart disease because they don't make enough estrogen.
2. Women with POI are unlikely to become pregnant again. Good news is that they may be able to have a child by using donated eggs.

PUTTING ANOVULATION IN PERSPECTIVE

The reasons why women don't ovulate every month are various and varied. Some are associated with specific stages of a woman's life, such as adolescence, pregnancy, breastfeeding, or the pre-menopausal period. More short-lived variables include the withdrawal from the pill or other hormone replacement therapy, stress, illness, weight gain, exercise, and travel.

Finally, there are those who are afflicted by more serious health issues. Understanding anovulatory cycles in their proper context is critical to their success. It's easy to take things for granted when everything goes according to plan. However, if you and your doctor suspect that you have a major medical problem, your charting will aid in the right diagnosis.

Many reproductive disorders can be treated with natural therapies, such as anovulation and irregular periods, which can be caused by a hormonal imbalance that can be remedied. Regardless, it's a good idea to consult with a doctor to be sure nothing more serious is going on.

FERTILITY AWARENESS AND ANOVULATION

When you're not ovulating, it's important to remember that you're still in your pre-ovulatory phase, and you should treat every day as if you were. The restrictions for using Fertility Awareness for contraception during anovulation are more complex, so keep that in mind if you're thinking of using it. The difficulty of this depends on your own anovulatory pattern.

12

Birth Control With Oral Contraceptives

Oral contraceptives that include modest amounts of hormones similar to those your body produces during the menstrual cycle are called birth control pills. Taking birth control pills prevents pregnancy because the hormones in the pills prevent an egg from being released from the ovary. A fertilized egg's ability to the implant may be hindered by several birth control medicines, which modify the uterine lining temporarily.

There are 28 days of birth control pills in a box, one pill for each day of the cycle. Depending on the pill, you normally take a birth control pill at the same time every day. You're less likely to become pregnant as a result of this since it keeps certain hormones up. When it comes to birth control, there are several options. It's possible to get pregnant while taking birth control tablets if you're sexually active.

Pregnancy-preventative medication that is used orally is called oral contraceptives. These contraceptives have a success rate of around 91%, according to the Food and Drug Administration (or a failure rate of 9 percent). To evaluate whether birth control pills are suitable for you, discover how they work, what side effects they may have, and other pertinent facts.

TYPES OF BIRTH CONTROL PILLS

Combination pills

The hormones estrogen and progesterone are synthetically generated in combination tablets (called progestin in its synthetic form). The menstrual cycle is regulated by estrogen.

During the middle of your cycle, your estrogen levels are at their highest, and at their lowest, during your menstrual cycle. After ovulation, progesterone thickens the endometrium to prepare the uterus for pregnancy. Ovulation is also prevented by high doses of progesterone.

In a 28-pack, you can get combination pills. The majority of pills in each cycle contain hormones since they are active. Other pills are inactive, meaning they do not contain hormones. Tablets for combination therapy are available in a variety of shapes and sizes.

- **Monophasic pills.** In a one-month cycle, these are given out. You receive the same hormone dosage from each active pill. During the final week of your cycle, you have the option of taking or skipping the inactive pills without affecting your period's timing.
- **Multiphasic pills.** These are given out in cycles of one month and contain varying amounts of hormones at each stage of the cycle. During the final week of your cycle, you have the option of taking or skipping the inactive pills without affecting your period's timing.
- **Extended-cycle pills.** Typically, these are given out every 13 weeks. 12 weeks are spent taking active tablets. You can take or not take the inactive pills during the last week of the cycle and still get your period. As a result,

you will only have menstruation three to four times each year at the most.

Brand-name combination pills include the following:

- Yaz
- Yasmin
- Velivet
- Seasonique
- Seasonale
- Ortho Tri-Cyclen
- Ortho-Novum
- Low-Ogestrel
- Ocella
- Natazia
- Loestrin
- Levora
- Kariva
- Estrostep Fe
- Enpresse
- Beyaz
- Azurette

Progestin-only pills

Only synthetic progesterone (progestin) is contained in progestin-only pills. The term "minipill" refers to this sort of pill. Heavy menstrual bleeding may be lessened with the use of solely progestin-containing tablets. There are those who may benefit from them, such as those who cannot take estrogen due to health issues or other factors, including a history of cardiovascular or circulatory problems such as stroke, migraines with aura, or deep vein thrombosis and / or heart disease.

In addition, if you're over 35 and smoke, you should avoid estrogen because it can raise your risk of blood clotting. Progestin-only pills ensure that the whole course of medication is taken. It's possible to get pregnant when taking progestin-only pills because there are no inactive pills.

Prescription-strength progestin-only medicines include:

- Ortho Micronor
- Nor-QD
- Jencycla
- Heather
- Errin
- Camila

ADVANTAGES AND DISADVANTAGES OF ORAL CONTRACEPTIVE

A woman's health can be jeopardized throughout pregnancy and childbirth. The non-contraceptive health benefits of contraceptives, which couples take to prevent conception, outweigh their own health concerns. Making an informed decision necessitates knowledge of the associated risks and advantages. By preventing pregnancies as well as reducing the risk of endometrial and ovarian cancer, as well as protecting against acute pelvic inflammation, oral contraceptives are among the most effective methods of preventing unwanted pregnancies. However, oral contraceptives have been linked to an increased risk of heart disease. IUDs are a reliable method of birth control, but they can raise the risk of infection for those women who are already predisposed to infection. Compared to more effective methods of contraception, barrier methods of contraception offer some protection against sexually transmitted illnesses, such as HIV (HIV). In some countries, the non-contraceptive advantages and hazards of contraceptives are more important than in others because of the prevalence of the disorders they treat.

This portion of the chapter examines the efficacy and health effects of various forms of contraception. Despite the fact that each approach has its own set of psychological hazards and rewards, our focus is mostly on the biological repercussions of a method's use. Our goal is to give information on the direct health implications of contraceptive use rather than the indirect health effects of fertility control on women's health. In some countries, health officials downplay the health benefits of lower fertility because they fear the adverse health effects of the widespread use of modern contraceptives, especially in circumstances where medical supervision of contraceptive practice is limited. This analysis is particularly important.

Advantages of Oral Contraceptive (OC)

The risk of iron deficiency anemia is reduced in both current and former users of oral contraceptives. The decrease in menstrual flow and the resulting rise in iron stores may be to blame. Iron insufficiency is a common concern in underdeveloped countries; thus, this advantage could be especially beneficial in those areas.

Case-control and cohort studies show that oral contraceptive use reduces the likelihood of developing benign breast disease. There is a higher relative risk of fibrocystic illness, fibroadenoma, and undiagnosed breast lumps for women who have used oral contraceptives for more than two years than for women who have not. Former users of oral contraceptives who haven't taken them in over a year don't continue to have this lower risk. Current oral contraceptive formulations may not have a protective effect against benign breast disease because of their high progestin content.

Several studies have connected oral contraceptive usage to a reduced prevalence of functioning ovarian cysts. This may be because ovulation has been suppressed. Oral contraceptives appear to offer some protection against uterine fibroids as well, and this protection appears to increase with time spent on the pill. Oral contraceptives' preventive effect against fibroids may be linked to the progestin's ability to alter the action of circulating estrogens, which may stimulate the production of fibroids.

PID, a prominent cause of female infertility, has been associated with oral contraceptive usage in various studies undertaken in both developed and developing countries. According to these researches, oral contraceptive use reduces cancer risk by an average of 40%. Oral contraceptives may alter the cervical mucus, preventing harmful organisms from rising into the upper vaginal tract; alternatively, oral contraceptives may limit monthly blood flow, thereby decreasing the quantity of media available for bacterial growth. Most studies of oral contraceptives and PID have been conducted in hospitals, which may not be applicable to women who are asymptomatic or who have PID that does not necessitate hospitalization. For example, oral contraceptives may provide protection against gonorrhea, a common cause of severe PID that necessitates hospitalization, whereas oral contraceptive use may provide little or no protection against other bacterial etiologies that cause less severe PID, such as chlamydia.

To reduce the chance of ectopic pregnancy, oral contraceptives are extremely effective at inhibiting ovulation. Current oral contraceptive users are ten times less likely to have an ectopic pregnancy than women who do not use the procedure (Ory and the Women's Health Study, 1981; Gray, 1984) based on extensive case-control studies. Because rural women in underdeveloped countries face a high risk of death from ectopic pregnancies, this consequence is of special importance.

In addition to reducing the incidence of endometrial and ovarian cancer, the usage of oral contraceptives is beneficial. Endometrial cancer risk has been reduced in a number of epidemiological studies. CASH (Cancer and Steroid Hormone) study undertaken in the United States indicated a 40% reduction in endometrial cancer risk, even after oral contraceptive use had ceased, and the effect increased with the total period of pill use. Although the pill's long-term effects on past users aren't fully understood, progestin in the pill appears to negate estrogen's carcinogenic effect on the endometrium.

It also revealed a 40% lower incidence of ovarian cancer in the CASH research (Centers for Disease Control and National Institute of Child Health and Human Development, 1987a, 1987b). These findings have been backed up by other epidemiological investigations. This protection may be provided by suppressing both ovulation and the hormone gonadotropin production. It is significant that independent epidemiological studies consistently show that the pill protects women from endometrial and ovarian cancer. True biological effect would be consistent with such constancy, it would seem.

Disadvantages of Oral Contraceptive

Cardiovascular Diseases

For the most part, research on oral contraceptive use and cardiovascular disease has occurred in industrialized countries, where cardiovascular disease is the main cause of mortality. In poor nations, the prevalence of these disorders is lower; hence, the impact of oral contraceptive use on its occurrence may be less significant than in industrialized countries.

When it comes to cardiovascular disease, oral contraceptive usage puts you at greater risk for heart attack, stroke, and venous thromboembolism, to name just a few. Older women over the age of 30 and women who smoke cigarettes or have other cardiovascular risk factors are most at risk from unfavorable cardiovascular effects from oral contraceptive use. Women who use both estrogen and progestins appear to have an increased risk of cardiovascular disease. Moreover, recent low-dose formulations may reduce the danger significantly.

In the case of thrombosis, a blood-clot obstruction in the vein occurs. It's possible for a clot to go from one place to another, such as the lungs or the brain, causing thrombosis. Death and illness are often linked to it. There is, however, a higher risk for present oral contraceptive users, although this risk does not remain among previous users and is unrelated to the length of time spent on oral contraceptives. There is an increased risk of both superficial and deep vein thrombosis if the estrogen level of the oral contraceptive is higher. VTE in pill users is not linked to cigarette smoking, at least in the short term. Increases in venous thromboembolism may be caused by estrogenic effects or blood clotting factors that make blood more coagulable.

In terms of oral contraceptive-related deaths, myocardial infarction and stroke are the two most common causes of death.

Age and other cardiovascular risk factors, such as smoking, hypertension, and diabetes, have a significant impact on the risk. Annual myocardial infarction risk increases from roughly 4 cases per 100,000 nonsmoking oral contraceptive users aged 30 to 39 to 185 cases per 100,000 heavy oral contraceptive smokers aged 40 to 44 due to current use of oral contraceptive. This is due to current oral contraceptive use. It has been discovered that current oral contraceptive use modestly raises blood pressure in the majority of females, which may be a contributing factor to the development of MI and stroke in current oral contraceptive users. Overt hypertension is three-to-sixfold more likely in women who use oral contraceptives, and this risk rises with age and duration of use. We must keep in mind that these dangers are related to the comparatively large dosages used back then, as well as patterns of use in connection to things like age and smoking.

Metabolic Effects

Myocardial infarction may be linked to metabolic alterations as a result of the use of oral contraceptives. The increase in HDL-cholesterol (high-density lipoprotein) caused by estrogens appears to be a beneficial impact. Progesterone can either raise or lower HDL cholesterol or have no impact on it at all, depending on the kind. A combination of estrogen and progestin doses affects HDL-cholesterol levels in a variety of ways.

However, most women's glucose tolerance was found to be reduced by the current usage of oral contraceptives, but this reduction was minor and unrelated to how long they had been taking them. The oral contraceptives' estrogen content has a direct bearing on this decline.

Neoplastic Diseases

Breast cancer, cervical cancer, endometrial cancer, and ovarian cancer are the most worrisome types of neoplasia for oral contraceptive users. For the most part, there are two reasons for this. First and foremost, these diseases are substantial causes of death and morbidity, notably in industrialized countries where breast cancer is prevalent and in poor countries where cervical cancer is prevalent. To begin with, the endocrine system is responsible for the development of these three organs, and numerous studies have shown that hormonal factors, such as menarche age and the age at which a woman gives birth for the first time, influence her risk of developing neoplastic disorders. A potential carcinogen or anti-carcinogen for these organs must therefore be carefully examined by any factor that affects hormones. In addition, the human papillomavirus (HPV), which causes cervical cancer, can be reduced with contraception.

The research of probable links between oral contraceptive usage and certain tumors is complicated by methodological issues. As a result of these issues, it may be difficult to evaluate factors that may affect the effects of oral contraceptives, such as the age at first pregnancy for breast cancer and the number of sexual partners for cervical cancer. In reality, some studies have found no correlation between Oral contraceptive use and breast and cervical cancer risk, while others have shown an increase. Unlike other health concerns, the discussion of breast and cervical cancer has taken on an urgency due to its high prevalence among women. Many countries' family planning programs lack the resources to appropriately monitor and respond to these malignancies. Many underdeveloped countries do not routinely undertake Papanicolaou (Pap) screening, for example, despite its commonplaceness in wealthier countries. Other malignancies seem to be less affected by oral contraceptive usage than endometrial and ovarian cancers.

It's debatable whether or not oral contraceptive use increases one's risk of developing breast cancer. Over the course of eight years, researchers in eight different parts of the United States worked on the Cancer and Steroid Hormone Study, the biggest study of its kind (Centers for Disease Control and National Institute of Child Health and Human Development, 1986). Regardless of the time of usage or oral contraceptive formulation, this investigation demonstrated no elevated risk of breast cancer in pill users. In fact, even women who are known to be at high risk for breast cancer, such as those who have had previous benign breast disease or a family history of the disease, were unaffected by the use of oral contraceptives. There is a lot of debate about long-term oral contraceptive use, early use, and use prior to full-term pregnancy. Premenopausal breast cancer was found to be more common in women who began taking oral contraceptives (oral contraceptives) with high levels of estrogen before the age of 25. Researchers showed that the risk of breast cancer quadrupled among women who had taken long-term oral contraceptives before having their first child. Though Pike and McPherson's analysis of the CASH data was repeated, a new examination of the data from the CASH trial indicated that very long-term oral contraceptive use might decrease the age of breast cancer detection for some nulliparous women without having a significant effect on the overall population.

The incidence of breast cancer, particularly premenopausal breast cancer, is extremely low among women in underdeveloped nations. In the aggregate, there is probably no significant increase in risk, even in tiny, select subgroups. As McPherson and colleagues (1983) note, the risk of breast cancer may not become apparent until 20 years after a person's first use of oral contraceptive, which means researchers may not be able to identify such a link at this time. Even in women who began using CASH at a young age, the CASH trial found no elevated risk of breast cancer in the 10 to 15 years following use. According to epidemiological research, oral contraceptives do not raise the risk of breast cancer, and any increase that may exist for some subgroups of women is not significant. In addition, the differences between research show that there may be methodological issues in the investigation of this complicated disease.

According to current statistics, cervical cancer is the most frequent malignancy among women in developing nations. Cervical cancer and oral contraceptive use have yet to be linked in a way that can be conclusively proven. No higher risk has been reported in several of the major epidemiological studies; however, there has been a considerable rise in risk in some subgroups. It was found that long-term use of oral contraceptives increases the risk of developing cancer, but the World Health Organization's 1985a study included many developing countries and had serious methodological flaws, such as the detection bias that results from more frequent screening of oral contraceptive users than nonusers and differences in sexual behavior between users and non-users. These methodological issues have been addressed in more recent studies, but the results are still inconclusive. While long-term oral contraceptive usage or use by specific subgroups of women may increase the risk of cervical dysplasia or cancer, the total risk is probably not greatly increased by oral contraceptives. Cervical neoplasia is more common among women who use oral contraceptives, according to two large cohort studies conducted in the United Kingdom. A significant finding of the debate over these data is the value of Pap screenings in preventing cervical cancer that spreads to other organs.

Melanoma, the most common form of skin cancer, has been linked to oral contraceptives; however, the link is weak and may be due to changes in sunshine exposure. Particularly among women who have used long-term, some research implies a rise in this population. There is a minimal attributable risk for public health policy in poor nations due to the rarity of this cancer.

Recent case-control studies have shown that long-term oral contraceptive users are more likely to develop hepatocellular carcinoma (liver cancer). Because of their limited sample sizes and methodological issues, these studies may have been prejudiced. Attributable risk for hepatocellular carcinoma is quite low in industrialized countries due to its rarity. Many developing countries, particularly those where chronic hepatitis B is prevalent, have a substantially higher incidence of the disease. Oral contraceptive use, hepatitis B, and liver cancer are all unknown to us. Three developing countries are being studied by the World Health Organization to answer the question.

A rare, benign growth of the liver known as a hepatocellular adenoma (HCA) has been linked to oral contraceptive use. HCA can induce intra-abdominal bleeding and even death if left untreated. An estimated 8% of patients die as a result of their injuries. Women who have taken oral contraceptives for at least five years have an extremely low risk of developing HCA, which is estimated to be two cases per 100,000 users per year.

Other Effects

Pregnant women who take oral contraceptives are more likely to suffer from gallbladder disease (Royal College of General Practitioners, 1982). however, the evidence supporting this claim is scant. Gall bladder disease may be more common in oral contraceptive users, according to early research (Boston Collaborative Drug Surveillance Program, 1974; Royal College of General Practitioners, 1982). Research conducted in the United Kingdom, where gallbladder illness was first linked to oral contraceptive use, has not been able to confirm this link.

Extensive research has been done on the impact of pre-and post-pregnancy hormonal contraceptive use on pregnancy outcomes. Many studies show no increased risks from synthetic steroids in utero at the doses used for contraception, but there are a few reports of negative side effects. Several comprehensive reviews of the literature have concluded that synthetic steroids used for contraception have no significant negative effects on fetal growth or development.

Mothers who are nursing have been demonstrated to be affected by the estrogen component of combination oral contraceptives, even at modest doses. Breastfeeding mothers can safely utilize progestin-only contraceptives like the minipill and long-acting methods described below because they have no effect on milk production (World Health Organization, 1981). In spite of the fact that the pill passes on synthetic hormones to suckling babies, no negative consequences have been found. The use of hormonal contraceptives before or during pregnancy has been linked in certain studies to an increased risk of birth abnormalities. Most research investigations, on the other hand, find no evidence of an elevated risk of harmful consequences on fetal development or growth.

HOW BIRTH CONTROL PILLS WORK

It is possible to take a combination tablet in two ways. Preventing ovulation is the first benefit. An egg will not be released each month because of this. This thickens your cervical mucus, which helps sperm travel to your uterus and fertilizes an egg in the process of taking these pills. The thicker mucus functions as a barrier to keep sperm from reaching the uterus.

However, progestin-only tablets may have a wide range of consequences. These drugs thicken cervical mucus and thin the endometrium. The endometrium refers to the uterine lining into which egg implants following fertilization. A thinner lining makes it more difficult for an egg to implant, preventing the development of a pregnancy. Pills that contain solely progestins may also prevent ovulation.

DECIDING ON THE BEST BIRTH CONTROL PILLS TO USE

Every person isn't a good candidate for every type of medicine. Consult your physician to find out which drug is best for your particular condition. Consider the following when making a decision:

- Your menstruation symptoms. When it comes to excessive bleeding, a progestin-only birth control tablet may be the best option for you.
- Whether or not you're nursing. If you're presently breastfeeding, you may want to avoid taking birth control pills that include estrogen.
- Your heart's health. Progestin-only birth control may be recommended if you've had a history of stroke, blood clots, and deep vein thrombosis.
- Other long-term health issues you may be dealing with. For women with chronic health conditions, such as

active breast or endometrial cancer, migraines with aura, or heart disease, oral contraception may not be the best option. Consult your physician and provide a complete medical history.

- As well as other medications you might be taking. Combination birth control may not be an option for you if you're using antibiotics or herbal medicines like St. John's Wort. It's possible that birth control pills will conflict with certain antiviral treatments or epileptic meds, and vice versa.

WHAT TO DO WHEN YOU FORGET TO TAKE YOUR BIRTH CONTROL PILLS

If you forget to take your birth control pill, use a contraceptive sponge, condom, or diaphragm with spermicide as a substitute. If you miss your pill at the wrong time during your cycle, your chances of getting pregnant go substantially.

If you skip one pill

It is recommended that you take the missed or late combo tablet as soon as you are aware of it, according to CDC guidelines.

- Continue to take the balance of your medication as scheduled (even if it means taking two pills on the same day). There's no need for any other methods of birth control.
- Even if the pills were missing early in your cycle or in the last week of your previous cycle, you could consider emergency contraception (except for ulipristal Ella).
- For missed medicines, always follow the instructions in your package insert. When in doubt, ask your doctor.

If you miss two pills

Take the most recent combination pill as soon as you remember if you miss more than 48 hours. Other medications that may have been missed should be thrown away.

- To minimize confusion, take your remaining prescriptions at the same time each day. While it may initially cause you to feel sick, the effects of taking two medications together will rapidly fade. Use condoms or avoid sex until you've taken your hormone pills for seven days in a row, whichever comes first.
- For 28-day pill packs, days 15–21 correspond to the last week of hormonal pills. If you missed any of these pills, it is advisable to bypass the hormone-free period by taking the remaining hormonal tablets in your current pack and beginning a new pack the following day. If you can't start a new pack right away, use a backup method of contraception (like condoms) or wait to engage in sexual activity until you've taken the hormone tablets in your new pack for seven days in a row.
- As long as the first week of hormonal pills was missed and unprotected sexual intercourse occurred within the previous five days, emergency contraception should be considered (with the exception of Ella). When the time is right, this can be brought up at other points.
- For missed medicines, always follow the instructions in your package insert. When in doubt, ask your doctor.

The estrogen and progestin combo tablet work best when taken at the same time each day. It is imperative that you take the progestin-only pills (mini-pills) at the same time each day (no more than 3 hours late). As a result, you will have a better chance of getting pregnant if you miss one of your daily pills.

Call your doctor if you miss three consecutive doses of a combo medication. It's possible that you'll have to switch to a new birth control technique while continuing to use your old one.

REMEMBER: Taking birth control pills is one of the most common ways to avoid pregnancy. Between 2015 and 2017, over 13.9% of women in the United States used oral contraceptives, which are also known as birth control tablets. The effectiveness of birth control pills is 99.7 percent when used correctly. Why are they so effective?

Progestin is the most common synthetic steroid hormone found in birth control pills, but some contain both progestin and estrogen. It is thought that these hormones inhibit the release of FSH and LH from the pituitary gland in the female body. Ovulation—the release of a mature egg from the female ovary—is stimulated by the production of estrogen from the ovaries, which is generally triggered by FSH and LH. The chances of ovulation, and thus sperm cell fertilization, are greatly lowered when FSH and LH are suppressed. If an egg is ovulated, progestin-only birth control pills thicken the cervix's mucus, preventing sperm from reaching the egg.

Menstrual cramps can be relieved with the help of birth control pills, which are often used to prevent pregnancy. This is because the body's prostaglandin levels are decreased by birth control pills. During pregnancy, the production of prostaglandins, which generate contractions in the uterine muscles, might result in cramping.

13

Foolproof Guides To Natural Birth Control Without Chemicals Or Devices

To avoid getting pregnant, women can utilize natural birth control, which does not include taking medication or using a contraceptive device. Observations of a woman's menstrual cycle and body have informed these theories.

In order to avoid unwanted pregnancies, natural birth control techniques may be used. Contraceptive methods that rely on nature are among the oldest. It is common for natural birth control to be free and without any physical adverse effects. This may lead to unplanned pregnancies; thus, caution should be exercised while using these procedures.

To be effective, a natural method of birth control requires that you be fully dedicated to it. Discipline and self-discipline are required to use these strategies. Being in a committed relationship where you and your partner can openly communicate and work together is also beneficial.

ABSTINENCE

A person is said to be abstinent if they do not engage in any form of sexual activity with another person. Pregnancy and sexually transmitted illnesses are prevented to the fullest extent possible by this procedure (STIs). Abstinence is a personal choice, but it can only succeed in a committed relationship if both partners are on board with it. Abstinence might be tough at times. It may be easier to keep to a decision if you have precise reasons for making it.

People's definitions of abstinence might vary widely. All forms of sexual intercourse, including vaginal, anal, and oral sex, must be avoided in order to achieve full sexual abstinence.

Abstinence may be referred to as a lack of vaginal intercourse but not as a complete lack of sexual activity. An "outercourse" is sexual activity that does not result in pregnancy, on the other hand. The following are some examples of an outercourse:

- Kissing
- Massage
- Masturbation
- Dry humping (clothes on)
- Anal sex
- Oral sex

Outercourse is just as efficient as abstinence in preventing pregnancy. However, it is possible for sperm to reach the vagina and fertilize an egg, resulting in pregnancy, if they touch the vulva during outercourse activities. Nonvaginal intercourse, such as anal sex and oral sex, can still transmit STIs, contrary to popular belief.

Abstinence to other people is abstaining from sex during the time of the month when they are most likely to conceive. "Periodic abstinence" is the ideal term to describe this strategy of natural family planning. Contrary to popular belief, complete cessation of sexual relations is not a guarantee against becoming pregnant.

Advantages of Abstinence

Abstaining from sex can be for a variety of reasons, including the desire to avoid pregnancy and sexually transmitted infections, religious convictions, medical considerations, and more. Abstinence from sexual activity has various rewards, no matter why you do it.

- It has no medical or hormonal adverse effects;
- It is 100 percent efficient in avoiding unwanted pregnancies and STIs.
- There is no cost to use it.

Disadvantages of Abstinence

- It has no medical or hormonal adverse effects;
- It is 100 percent efficient in avoiding unwanted pregnancies and STIs.
- There is no cost to use it.

Talking to Your Partner

Having a discussion with your spouse about your decision to abstain is essential if you've decided to do so. A spouse who doesn't know why you made a decision may interpret it as a personal attack. It is much simpler to refrain from having sex for an extended period of time when both partners are on board with it.

Planned Parenthood provides the following suggestions for starting the conversation:

- Having faith in your choice.
- Being open and honest with yourself and others about your decision to abstain.

- Talking to your partner ahead of time, rather than in the middle of a sexual encounter.
- Reminding yourself and your partner that your decision may evolve over time.

WITHDRAWAL

The act of withdrawing one's penis from the vagina before ejaculating is known as withdrawal. Because some people, when aroused, eject pre-ejaculate fluid, which may include sperm, this may not be a viable natural birth control approach. To fertilize an egg, one sperm is all that is needed; therefore, these sperm are released into the vagina.

Withdrawal is another technique that necessitates total self-control. To successfully remove your penis, you must have a precise sense of timing. The effectiveness of this approach as a birth control strategy is about 78%. Every year, around 1 in 5 people who use withdrawal become pregnant.

EFFECTIVENESS OF THE WITHDRAWAL METHOD

The withdrawal method is sometimes performed during sex in order to reduce the likelihood of becoming pregnant. The "pullout method" or "coitus interruptus" are other names for this technique.

If you're attempting to prevent getting pregnant, this is a dangerous strategy. When done correctly, this procedure carries a 4-percent probability of becoming pregnant. The pullout procedure will result in four pregnancies for every 100 couples. Keeping in mind that this figure only applies to couples that follow the process step-by-step is critical.

USING THE PULL OUT METHOD CORRECTLY

This strategy demands a lot of self-control and time to be used correctly. Ejaculation cannot be delayed or stopped once a man has reached the point of no return. This is essential if you want to get out of there when it's time. When it comes to getting pregnant, it doesn't matter if your spouse has tremendous self-control.

Without any additional means of birth control, using the withdrawal method is dangerous. It's still possible to become pregnant due to the discharge of pre-ejaculate semen prior to ejaculation, even if your intended partner pulled out. If you're ovulating, the sperm in this minuscule amount of semen can help you conceive. Ovulation is the process of releasing an egg into the uterus.

It is also possible to get pregnant by spilling semen or pre-ejaculate on the vulva (the exterior opening of the vagina). The pullout approach also has the drawback of failing to provide protection against sexually transmitted illnesses (STIs).

BENEFITS OF THE WITHDRAWAL METHOD

When it comes to contraception, the withdrawal method is among the most dangerous. There are some advantages to utilizing it nonetheless. The following is an example:

- Both parties find it easy and convenient to pull out.
- When no other method of birth control is available, it can be utilized.
- Using this approach has not been associated with any medical or hormonal negative effects.
- There is no need for a prescription.
- There is no cost to utilize it.

- It can improve the effectiveness of other methods of birth control when used in conjunction with them.

RISKS OF PULLING OUT

Using this form of birth control is extremely risky. Even if it's your only type of birth control, this is especially true. The following is an example:

- A high risk of pregnancy.
- It does not protect against STIs.
- It is very easy to use wrongly, especially for youths and sexually inexperienced males.
- If you don't have a lot of self-discipline or experience, it's not going to work.
- If a man experiences premature ejaculation, he should not take this product.

REDUCING THE RISKS OF THE PULLOUT METHOD

If you want to avoid getting pregnant, consider using another kind of birth control, such as:

Condoms

The proper way to put on a condom is essential if you're relying on it for contraception or protection from STIs (sexually transmitted illnesses). Even while it may appear simple, it's easy to misplace it. Using male condoms as a form of birth control is one of the most prevalent methods. Learn how to utilize them if you're male or have sex with biological males.

- *Check the Expiration Date*

To get the most out of a condom, make sure it's still usable before using it. Before using a condom, always verify its expiration date. The latex in condoms degrades if they are old or incorrectly stored. This raises the likelihood that the condom won't be as effective, which could result in an unwanted pregnancy or sexually transmitted infection. The packing should be in good condition, too. Even if the expiration date is on the packaging, throw it away if you find a hole or a rip.

- *Feel for the Air Bubble*

Feeling for an air bubble is another way to ensure that a condom packet is still fresh. Condoms are protected from damage by an air bubble in the box. Its existence indicates that the condom's package is intact and that the condom is safe to use. Gently squeeze the packet between your thumb and first finger to find the bubble.

- *Open the Package Carefully*

Although the foil packets that condoms come in are very simple to open, extreme caution should be exercised when doing so. Wash your hands first. Foreplay fluids can contaminate the condom; thus, this is especially crucial if you have your hands dirty. Open the package by carefully tearing it open from the corner or edge (most packaging indicates where you should tear). The condom and the wrapper can be ripped if you use your nails, scissors, or any other sharp object.

- *Find the Correct Side of the Condom*

Determine which side of the condom you'll be placing on your penis by holding it up to the light. This should be done on the outside rather than hidden inside. If necessary, you can check for this by unrolling the condom a little bit. This shouldn't necessitate you inserting your fingers into the condom. If you can comfortably roll the condom down over the penis, you have the correct side.

- *Make Room and Put the Condom On*

Place the condom's tip on the penis with the pads of your fingers. By doing so, you're ensuring that the fluid discharged during ejaculation has somewhere to go (climax). If you don't have it, the condom could break. As a bonus, this will keep the condom from becoming stale. The reservoir tip of most condoms is used for this function.

- *Unroll the Condom All the Way*

As soon as you've got the condom in place, unroll it to make sure it covers the whole penis shaft. Syphilis, for example, can be transmitted by skin-to-skin contact, and this will help lower the risk of transmission. It also reduces the risk of the condom slipping if it is rolled all the way down. The condom is too tiny if it doesn't completely cover the shaft of the penis or if it feels tight. It's more likely that a condom will fail if it's too little or too large.

- **Check for Trapped Air**

To determine whether or not the condom is filled with air, feel the tip. A broken condom is more likely to occur if the condom is left in this position. Place your hands around the penis and carefully smooth out the condom from the tip to the base. The tip of the condom can assist prevent this by being lubricated before use.

- **Hold the Condom When Withdrawing**

Immediately following ejaculation, condoms should be gently removed from the penis to prevent it from drooping. To restrict the ejaculate from spilling out, hold onto the base of the penis as it is pulled from the vagina, anus, or mouth. Close the open end of the condom with your fingers to keep it from sliding out of your partner's body. In the absence of this precaution, the condom may slip and leak.

- **Throw Away the Condom**

Instead of flushing condoms down the toilet, dispose of them properly. The pipelines can choke. To avoid leakage and a messy situation, wrap the condom in toilet paper or a paper towel. In addition, your personal information is better safeguarded this way.

REMEMBER: One of the most effective methods of pregnancy control and disease prevention is condom use. They must, however, be used correctly if they are to work well. Always verify the product's expiration date and packaging before opening it, and do it with caution. Leave space for ejaculate when putting it on, then unroll it so that the right side is facing out. When you've finished with your companion, dispose of the condom by holding it in place. Using a condom that is as effective as possible can be achieved by following these best practices.

FERTILITY AWARENESS METHODS

In order to figure out when you're most fertile, you have to keep an eye on your body using fertility awareness approaches. You can avoid having unprotected intercourse around the time of ovulation if you use condoms. Recording changes in your body (such as your basal body temperature or cervical mucus) can help you anticipate when you'll ovulate naturally.

You must be willing to keep track of your fertility signs in order to succeed. Afterward, you and your partner must agree to refrain from intercourse for five days before ovulation, as sperm can remain in the reproductive canal for up to five days.

The Billings, Symptothermal, and Standard Days techniques all fall under the category of fertility awareness. Fertility iPhone Apps can also help you keep track of your body's changes. A book like "Taking Charge of Your Fertility: The Definitive Guide to Natural Birth Control" might help explain how to undertake natural family planning.

For every 100 couples who use fertility awareness approaches, about 12 to 24 of them will conceive each year, which is only a 76% to 88% success rate.

OUTERCOURSE

It's a phrase that covers a wide range of sexual acts, and it can be used in a variety of situations. Frotage, tribadism, and other non-penetrational forms of sexual body rubbing are commonly described as this. Sharing sex fantasies and sexual desires can also be included in this category.

A male partner thrusting his penis to orgasm between his partner's legs, breasts, butt cheeks, or other body parts in a simulation of intercourse is also known as outercourse. The absence of vaginal, oral, or anus penetration is, once again, the defining characteristic. "Dry humping" is a common term for this type of activity.

Outercourse vs. Abstinence

The term "outercourse" can refer to any sexual act that does not involve vaginal penetration and hence carries a low chance of pregnancy in some groups. Abstinence and outercourse are comparable in this respect. Abstinence is also defined in a variety of ways. Some people define abstinence as having no sex at all. Those who are opposed to getting pregnant see it as anything that doesn't allow them to do so. Be a result, abstinence and outercourse are often referred to as the same thing.

Outercourse may encompass oral and/or anal sex for those who define it simply in terms of pregnancy risk. This is not how most sex educators and sexuality experts use the term. Abstaining from oral and anal sex isn't considered abstinence by most sex educators. Nonetheless, there are many who disagree.

Advantages of Outercourse

Outercourse is a method by which some people engage in sexual activity with another person without running the danger of becoming pregnant. In that sense, it is really a very effective method. As long as heterosexual couples are mindful of the male partner ejaculating close to the vagina, the risk of getting pregnant is low. Outercourse couples are not in danger of pregnancy, regardless of whether they're male/female or male/female. Some couples who observe abstinence (before marriage or at some point in their relationship) may find outercourse a good alternative for sexual activity. Body stroking can be enjoyable and can lead to orgasm without breaking any religious rules. People whose sexual behaviors are restricted due to religious or other reasons may find this to be a delightful activity, of course.

People who aren't concerned about being pregnant or abstinent can also enjoy outercourse. Body massaging and other outercourse activities can be enjoyed as either a prelude or the centerpiece of a romantic encounter. Penetrative sex isn't something everyone is interested in. For others, the novelty of an outercourse is a welcome change of pace. It can be a delightful approach to get to know a new or long-time companion. Even for those who don't want to spend time discussing their sexual preferences, outercourse is a relatively safe option.

Disadvantages of Outercourse

Even though body rubbing is a low-risk activity, it is not a risk-free form of sexual activity. You may still be at risk for some sexually transmitted illnesses that pass from skin to skin even if you're not in a sexual relationship.

Condoms or other barriers can be used to make the outside world a safer place. It is also possible to participate in various outercourse activities while wearing garments. Outercourse, on the other hand, is a generally risk-free activity even when performed barefoot. Even though skin infections can be transferred, they provide a much lower risk than those spread by vaginal, oral, or anal sex. Even people with HIV utilize it as a risk-reduction strategy.

Negotiate your preferences and boundaries before getting into an out-of-body experience with a new companion. It's a good idea to make sure you and your partner are on the same page about what an outercourse is before embarking on one. The level of intimacy between the thighs, buttocks or other areas of the body is vastly different when the frottage is completely clothed.

Is it Possible for Outercourse to Lead to Intercourse?

Outercourse can, according to some, lead to intercourse as a negative side effect. True, a small amount of sexual pleasure might lead to a desire for more. Nevertheless, the notion that one activity inevitably leads to another is fraught with difficulty. It gives the impression that people have little control over their sexual orientation. Even if outercourse encourages you to desire intercourse, you may choose whether or not to engage in it. Even if you're not taking an exterior course, this is still true! Outercourse cannot be sexually fulfilling because intercourse involves a risk of it. It is possible. Sexual action isn't all about penetration. Without penetration, people can enjoy a satisfying sex life, sometimes without even removing their clothes!

CONTINUOUS BREASTFEEDING (LACTATIONAL AMENORRHEA METHOD)

For up to six months after giving birth, women can delay ovulation using the lactational amenorrhea method (constant breastfeeding). It works because the hormone required for milk production blocks the release of the ovulation-inducing hormone.

Using this approach for more than six months or if you have gotten your period since giving birth is not recommended.

Lactational amenorrhea is possible if the mother breastfeeds her infant at least once a day and once at night.

How Continuous Breastfeeding Works

Continuous breastfeeding after giving birth can be used as a means of contraception while breastfeeding. Your kid must be exclusively breastfed for LAM to work, which means no other liquids save your breast milk. Since ovulation can only occur when a mother is breastfeeding, it is possible to inhibit the release of the ovulation-inducing hormone by breastfeeding. When your body doesn't produce an egg each month, pregnancy is impossible.

Advantages of the Lactational Amenorrhea Method

Breastfeeding is a proven technique of birth prevention that is both safe and effective. The Lactational Method of Amenorrhea:

- There are no side effects.
- It's easy and cost-free.
- Does not need to be prescribed by a doctor or be under their care.
- It works immediately.
- After birth, bleeding is lessened thanks to this method.
- There is no need to plan sexual encounters ahead of time, allowing for greater sexual spontaneity (like a diaphragm, condom, sponge, spermicide, or female condom).

In addition to the benefits to your own health, the benefits to your child's health from breast milk are numerous. Among them are:

- Your baby will be more comfortable, and you will be able to form a stronger attachment with your child as a result.
- Allergic reactions are less likely, and asthma is less likely, as well.
- Some of your mother's antibodies can cross through and protect your baby from certain infections.
- It's essential to feed your infant only the highest-quality foods.

Disadvantages of the Lactational Amenorrhea Method

- There is no protection from sexually transmitted illnesses.
- You can only rely on it 6 months after giving birth
- Vaginal lubrication may be reduced as a result.
- In order to successfully breastfeed your child, you may have to put in some extra effort.
- Breastfeeding, according to some women, might make the breasts appear less sexy.

Can You Get Pregnant While Breastfeeding?

You should be aware, however, that the Lactational Amenorrhea Method is a viable method of birth control and that it has significant drawbacks.

- Breastfeeding as a method of contraception should only be relied upon if your period has not yet returned and it has been less than six months since you gave birth.
- Breastfeeding mothers may feel more secure using this method of contraception.

Effectiveness of the Lactational Amenorrhea Method

Breastfeeding can be an effective natural contraceptive method for up to six months following the birth of a child if your period has not yet returned.

- It is 95 percent effective for typical use.
- It is 98 percent effective for perfect use.

In the first six months of using LAM, 5 out of every 100 women will become pregnant, and less than 2 out of every 100 women will become pregnant with perfect use.

- Only women who exclusively breastfeed for the first six months after giving birth are eligible for the effectiveness rates.

REMEMBER: The following information is critical if you plan to use breast milk as a method of birth control and want to avoid becoming pregnant while doing so:

- You can only use breastfeeding as a method of contraception for the first six months after giving birth.
- Do not feed your baby anything other than breast milk during this time.
- It is recommended that you nurse your child at least four times a day and six times a night.
- Since giving birth to your child, you haven't had a monthly period.

You should not use LAM for more than six months or after having a period since the birth of your child. You'll have to switch to another kind of birth control by the time your child is six months old, even if you're exclusively breastfeeding (or if you get your period before this time).

You must nurse your child at least six times a day with both breasts and not substitute any other meal for breast milk in order for this strategy to function. In order to avoid pregnancy while breastfeeding, women who use LAM should do the following:

- Allow only 5 percent to 10 percent of supplemental feedings for the optimum contraceptive benefits for mothers and their newborns.
- For optimal results, mothers should feed their children every four hours during the day and every six hours at night.

Conclusion

One of the most perplexing and divisive issues facing women's health has been the debate over birth control, which has raged for decades. The United States, like many other countries, has a long history of enacting laws to restrict access to contraceptives. Because of Margaret Sanger's bravery in the early 1900s, condoms and diaphragms were first made legal and widely available in the United States.

In 1916, Sanger built the first birth control clinic in the United States in Brooklyn, New York, and was jailed and pursued as a result of printing newsletters calling for such access to the clinic. (Police shut down the clinic in an instant.) The American Birth Control League, a precursor to Planned Parenthood, had 37,000 members by the early 1920s as a result of her efforts. In the face of both legal challenges and hostility from the male-dominated medical establishment, the power of this and other organizations prevailed.

A few generations later, the emergence of the pill marked the most significant change in contemporary contraceptive history. The first really organized organization devoted to women's health was sparked by the difficulties women had in revealing its harmful side effects (many of which have now been rectified). A year after protesters disrupted a Senate hearing on the pill in 1969 because no women were called to testify about their own negative experiences with it, the Boston Women's Health Book Collective published the first mimeograph booklets of what soon evolved into the landmark tome *Our Bodies, Ourselves*, and this is no coincidence.

There was a backlash against the overuse of radical mastectomies for breast cancer and a desire for greater information about DES and its terrible consequences on a generation of girls born to mothers who had used it by the time abortion became legal in 1973. For many women, access to safe and effective contraceptive options is still one of the most important issues in women's health today, considering the well-publicized hazards of both the pill (and later the IUD) and the IUD itself.

Bibliography

"Contraception and Reproduction: Health Consequences for Women and Children in the Developing World," National Library of Medicine, accessed July 7, 2022, https://www.ncbi. nlm.nih.gov/books/NBK235069/.

Helen B., Betty, B., & Michael, G. (1980). Birth Control And Controlling Birth: Women-Centered Perspectives. Humana Press Inc.

Laura, E. (2010). In Our Control: The Complete Guide to Contraceptive Choices for Women. Seven Stories Press.

Ruth, T. (2003). Women, Hormones And The Menstrual Cycle. Allen & Unwin.

Toni, W. (2015). Taking Charge of Your Fertility: The Definitive Guide to Natural Birth Control, Pregnancy, Achievement, and Reproductive Health. HarperCollins Publisher.

"Your Guide to Birth Control Pills: Types, Effectiveness, and Safety," Healthline, accessed July 2, 2022, https://www. healthline.com/health/birth-control-pills#effectiveness.

"Types of Birth Control Pills (Oral Contraceptives)," Drugs.com, accessed July 10, 2022, https://www.drugs.com/article/birth-control-pill.html.